Neuro-Logic

Neuro-Logic

A Primer on Localization

Phillip L. Pearl, MD
William G. Lennox Chair and Director
Epilepsy and Clinical Neurophysiology
Boston Children's Hospital
Professor of Neurology
Harvard Medical School
Boston, MA

Formerly Division Chief, Neurology
Children's National Medical Center
Professor of Neurology, Pediatrics, and Music
The George Washington University School of Medicine and Health
Sciences and Columbian College of Arts and Sciences
Washington, DC

Helene A. Emsellem, MD
Clinical Professor of Neurology
The George Washington University School of Medicine
and Health Sciences
Washington, DC
Director, The Center for Sleep & Wake Disorders
Chevy Chase, MD

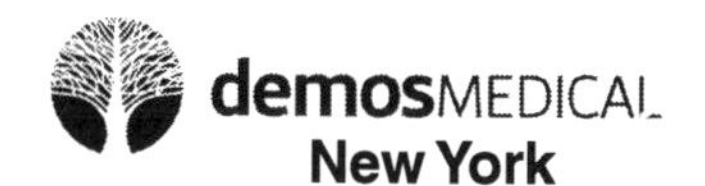

Visit our website at www.demosmedical.com

ISBN: 9781620700419
e-book ISBN: 9781617052071

Acquisitions Editor: Beth Barry
Compositor: Amnet

Medicine is an ever-changing science. Research and clinical experience are continually expanding our knowledge, in particular our understanding of proper treatment and drug therapy. The authors, editors, and publisher have made every effort to ensure that all information in this book is in accordance with the state of knowledge at the time of production of the book. Nevertheless, the authors, editors, and publisher are not responsible for errors or omissions or for any consequences from application of the information in this book and make no warranty, expressed or implied, with respect to the contents of the publication. Every reader should examine carefully the package inserts accompanying each drug and should carefully check whether the dosage schedules mentioned therein or the contraindications stated by the manufacturer differ from the statements made in this book. Such examination is particularly important with drugs that are either rarely used or have been newly released on the market.

Library of Congress Cataloging-in-Publication Data

Pearl, Phillip L., author.
Neuro-logic : a primer on localization / Phillip L. Pearl and Helene A. Emsellem.
p. ; cm.
Includes bibliographical references and index.
ISBN 978-1-62070-041-9 (print : alk. paper) — ISBN 978-1-61705-207-1 (e-book)
I. Emsellem, Helene A., author. II. Title.
[DNLM: 1. Central Nervous System. 2. Central Nervous System Diseases. 3. Neuropsychiatry—methods. 4. Peripheral Nervous System Diseases. 5. Peripheral Nervous System. WL 300]
RC346
616.8—dc23

2013043469

Printed in the United States of America by McNaughton & Gunn.
14 15 16 17 / 6 5 4 3 2

For Maurice and Betty Pearl, my first teachers; Melinda and Andrew, Adam, Suzanne, Natalie, and Caroline, my first students; Charles and Ann Tartaglia, for their insights; and Maria, for her support.

—Phillip L. Pearl, MD

To all of my students and patients—past, present, and future—who continue to challenge me with thoughtful questions and help me strive to find clear explanations.

—Helene A. Emsellem, MD

Contents

Contributors

Julia B. Frank, MD
Director, Medical Student Education in Psychiatry
Professor, Department of Psychiatry and Behavioral Sciences
The George Washington University School of Medicine and Health Sciences
Washington, DC

Lorin M. Scher, MD
Director, Emergency Psychiatry
Psychosomatic Medicine Service;
Health Sciences Assistant Clinical Professor
Department of Psychiatry & Behavioral Sciences
University of California, Davis, School of Medicine
Sacramento, California

Preface

Neuro-Logic: A Primer on Localization is for the student of clinical neurology—whether premed, medical student, resident, or beyond. This project began in our quest to provide a reasonably digestible syllabus for medical students and others taking preclinical courses that provide an introduction to clinical medicine.

An overriding goal was to prepare a clear and understandable format that could be mastered during a 2-week course, which was the duration used at George Washington University School of Medicine for neurology during the second-year introduction to clinical medicine course. It presupposes that students have (more or less) had their first-year medical school curriculum of neuroscience that includes neuroanatomy, neurophysiology, and neuroembryology. This book is written primarily for the student just embarking on clinical training who needs to put it all together—that is, the voluminous basic neuroscience information with the skills of the neurological examination, disease-based information, and what will be encountered on the wards and in the clinic. It should serve as a neurological foundation for the medical student or house officer who is confronted with learning how to examine the nervous system and interpret its diseases, whether in the lecture hall or the clinic.

This volume would also be appropriate for clinicians at all stages wishing to brush up on neurological training, and conceivably for undergraduate or graduate university students who want to amalgamate their work in neurosciences with the clinical arena. It has evolved from a series of lectures to a syllabus to its present form. The text is designed to instill both an understanding of the fundamentals of neurological localization and enough pertinent details to prove there really is life after the basic science years. The original course was under the direction of Dr. Emsellem; the course was then conducted by Dr. Pearl, who decided that the playful, cartoon-filled syllabus was too important to lose and instead should be preserved as a full-fledged book, replete with text and figures placed on the computer and revised many times over. Our colleagues in psychiatry, Drs. Frank and Scher, took on the challenge of contributing a chapter on psychiatry that could be applied to the same model and core mission: instructing the student of neurology with a localization-based understanding of the nervous system.

Special thanks go to the students and postgraduate physicians who reviewed portions of this manuscript as it was in preparation (listed chronologically based on their participation): Denise Wallis, Philip Capp, Ana Roche-Martinez, Georgann Ferrone, Lily Maltz, Ameeka Pannu, Regina DePietro, and Emily Barrios. We are grateful to Children's National child neurology fellows who reviewed the text during our localization course: Scott Demarest, MD and Jonathan Kurz, MD, PhD. Thank you to Demos editors Beth Barry and Lee Oglesby for helping this project come to fruition. Special acknowledgments are due to Veronica Reyes, Joseph Knight, and David Hutchinson, RN, for contributing their expertise in computer graphics.

This book was made possible by generous support from the Master Teacher Program in Medical Education at the Children's National Medical Center and the School of Education, The George Washington University School of Medicine, Washington, DC, and from the Delman Family Fund for Pediatric Neurology Research and Education.

Phillip L. Pearl, MD
Helene A. Emsellem, MD

1

Introduction to Localization: "Where's the Beef?"

Remember the television commercial where the unsuspecting but hungry diner peers into the hamburger bun and asks: "Where's the beef?" That's a big part of what neurologists do. Before the advent of CT (computed tomography) scans, MRIs (magnetic resonance imaging), and the other imaging modalities, physicians used the clinical approach to identify where in the nervous system the problem lay. Physicians had well-developed localization skills—they could tell where the lesion was. The classical neurologist laments that these localization skills seem to be atrophying. We have all become (overly) dependent on imaging tests and our friendly colleagues in neuroradiology who possess the answer to the age-old question in neurology: "Where is the lesion?"

However, imaging is not enough. Many neurological disease processes occur at a level lower than the resolution of current imaging technologies. It is imperative to know the patient's clinical presentation, which requires a careful history and neurological examination. Both entail well-honed skills. Then imaging findings must be correlated with the clinical data. The clinical information plus imaging findings together are both necessary to explain the patient's condition because sometimes there is a mismatch where the imaging does not explain the clinical presentation. This is the realm of the neurologist.

This primer demonstrates a logical approach to the nervous system that should serve the student throughout medical school rotations, postgraduate residency training, and medical practice during the lifelong learning task of evaluating patients with neurological problems.

2

The Central Nervous System: Brain and Cord

A. THE CEREBRAL HEMISPHERES: STARTING AT THE TOP

Case presentation: A high school senior interviewed for a summer job at the local factory. The building was aging and needed repairs. He told the boss he wanted to start at the top. When he reported for work the first day of summer, he was assigned to the roof.

Central nervous system (CNS)

- Brain
  - Cerebrum
  - Cerebellum
  - Brainstem
- Spinal cord

Peripheral nervous system (PNS)

- Nerve roots
- Ganglia
- Peripheral nerves
- Neuromuscular junctions
- Muscles
- Sensory receptors outside the brain and spinal cord

The central nervous system (CNS) is composed of the brain and spinal cord. The brain includes the cerebrum, cerebellum, and brainstem. The peripheral nervous system (PNS) includes all the nerve roots, ganglia, peripheral nerves, neuromuscular junctions, muscles, and sensory receptors outside of the brain and spinal cord. Many students and investigators study the nervous system because they are fascinated with this basic question of humanity: "How does the brain work?" This book begins with the study of the brain.

The brain is organized into the four lobes of each cerebral hemisphere, plus the basal ganglia, thalamus and hypothalamus (diencephalon), brainstem, and cerebellum. The lobes of each cerebral hemisphere are the frontal, parietal, temporal, and occipital lobes (Figure 2.1). There may be a newly classified lobe, the limbic lobe, to encompass deep, insulated tissue associated with the limbic system, which governs emotion and to some extent memory. Neuroanatomists have been discussing this new scheme for a long time. From embryological and evolutionary aspects, the most advanced part of the brain really is at the top—the cerebral cortex (telencephalon).

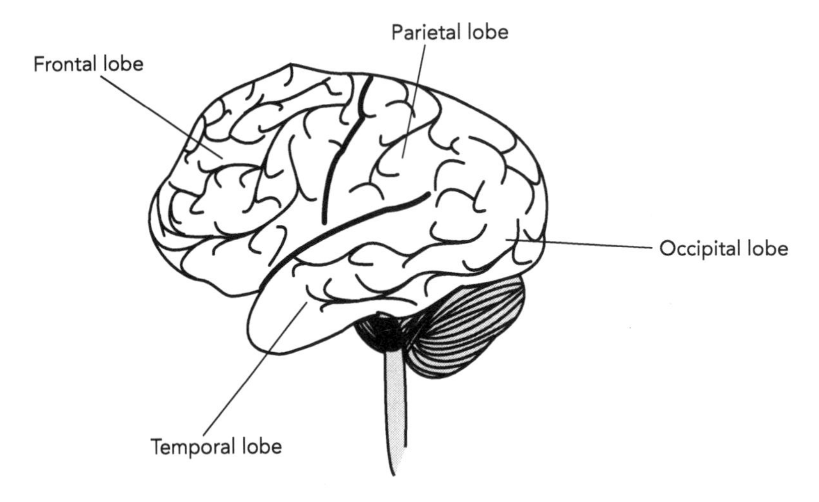

Figure 2.1 Overview of brain anatomy—the four lobes.

The function of the cerebral cortex is to provide an integrated assessment of incoming sensory information and generate appropriate motor responses. The location of a neurological abnormality, or so-called lesion, will determine what type of sensory or motor information is affected. In general, although there are widespread interacting networks throughout the brain, each lobe of the cerebral hemispheres is specialized to handle different functions:

Frontal Lobe: Motor and Higher Executive Functions
Parietal Lobe: Sensory Functions
Temporal Lobe: Hearing, Memory, and Language Comprehension
Occipital Lobe: Visual Perception

As an added attraction, the human brain is capable of storing links between experiences and the emotions they evoke, creating complex memories in which the original sensations or movements may be retrieved along with their meanings. A variety of classification schemes, based on microscopic appearance and function, exist for different regions of the cerebral cortex. The most widely known of these was published by Korbinian Brodmann at the turn of the 20th century. On the basis of histologic studies, Brodmann divided and labeled regions of the cortex according to similar cytoarchitectural features. Many of these regions proved to be functionally related and retain their numbered classifications. In this text a combined approach is used, studying the cortex in terms of the anatomically determined lobes and the Brodmann areas when applicable (Figure 2.2).

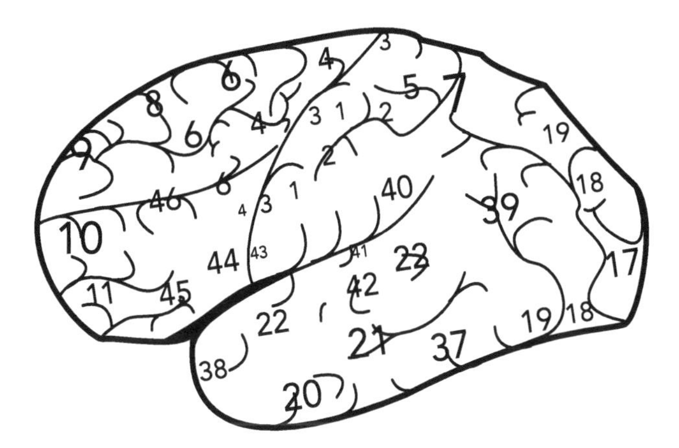

Figure 2.2 Brodmann areas of the brain.

1. Frontal Lobes

Motor strip

The motor strip occupies the precentral gyrus (Brodmann area 4) in the frontal lobe (Figure 2.2). It lies directly in front of (anterior to) the central sulcus, which divides the frontal and parietal lobes (Figure 2.3). Neurons responsible for innervation of all muscle groups lie along this strip in an anatomically determined fashion.

This topographical organization is represented by the homunculus, the little man who lives on top of the brain (Figure 2.4). He is best named "HAL," to commemorate the organization from head to arm to leg in a lateral to medial pattern. There is a homologous, but not identical, version over the main sensory strip of the parietal lobe (Brodmann areas 3, 1, and 2) that lies posterior to the central sulcus. Note the large cortical area devoted to the lips, tongue, face, and fingers (especially thumb). Evolution of the human brain had a role in allowing for very finely coordinated motor activity of these areas.

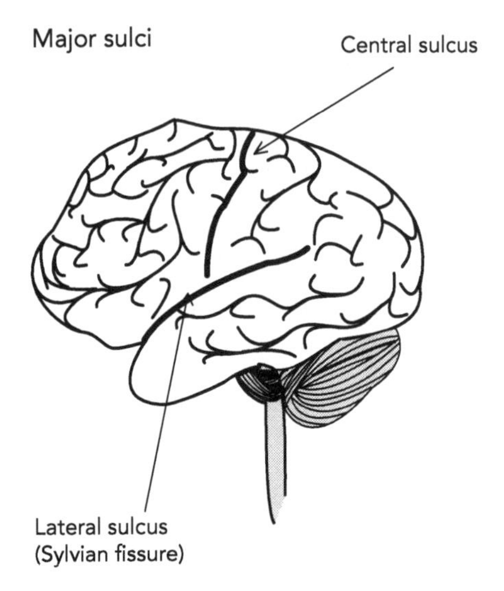

Figure 2.3 The frontal lobe is separated from the parietal lobe by the central sulcus, and from the temporal lobe beneath by the lateral sulcus, also known as the Sylvian fissure.

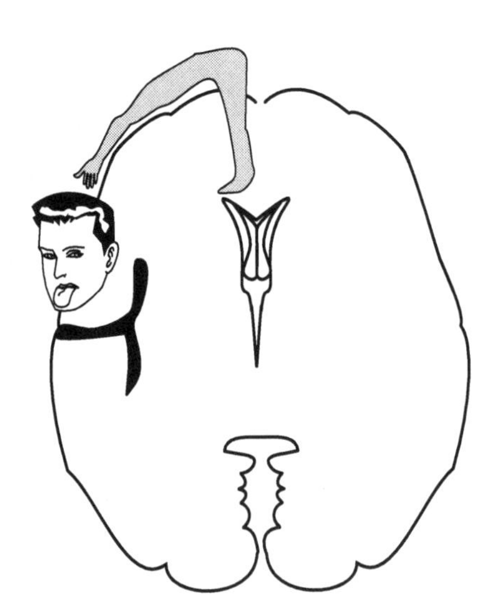

Figure 2.4 Monsieur Homunculus!

Vascular territories

The *blood supply* to the motor strip is shared by the anterior and middle cerebral arteries, arising from the internal carotid artery (Figure 2.5). The anterior cerebral artery (ACA) supplies most of the cortex on the anterior medial surface of the brain, from the frontal to the anterior parietal lobes. This covers

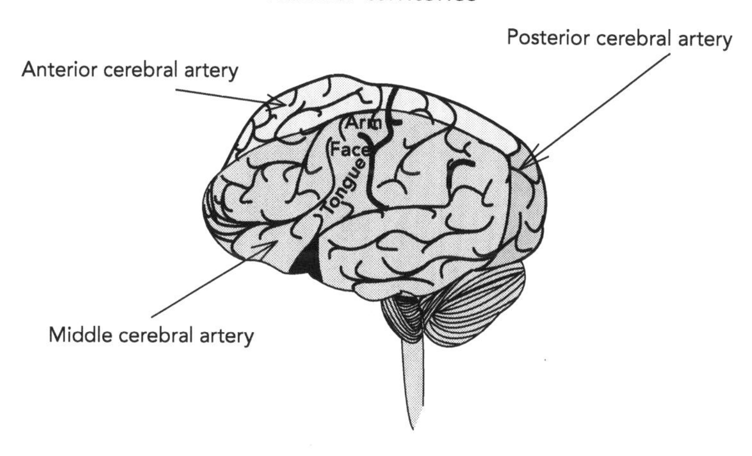

Figure 2.5 The anterior cerebral artery (ACA), middle cerebral artery (MCA), and posterior cerebral artery (PCA) are the major arteries supplying blood to the brain. The MCA and ACA are branches arising from the internal carotid artery and may be referred to as the "anterior circulation." The PCA is derived from the basilar artery or "posterior circulation."

the medial and inner surface of the frontal lobe. The motor strip involving the lower extremity is in this vascular distribution. The middle cerebral artery (MCA) supplies most of the cortex over the lateral convexity of the brain, and hence is responsible for perfusion of the cortex that innervates the arm, face, and tongue. The clinical manifestations of a cerebrovascular event thus can be understood based on the blood vessel(s) involved.

The primary motor tract extends from the motor strip in the cerebral cortex to the spinal cord. Hence, the corticospinal tract, as illustrated in Figure 2.6.

The pattern of motor symptoms that arise when the fibers of the corticospinal tract are disrupted varies depending on the level of the lesion. In a cortical lesion, there tends to be differential involvement of the extremities. If the cause of the disruption is a blockage of the anterior cerebral artery or a medial frontal lobe mass, then the leg will be affected dramatically, with only minimal weakness in the arm and no weakness in the face (all on the opposite side of the body). In contrast, in the more common infarction of the middle cerebral artery, the face and arm on the opposite side may be affected much more dramatically than the leg. If the entire carotid artery is occluded, then the face, arm, and leg may all be equally affected.

The fibers of the corticospinal tract descend from the cortex through the subcortical white matter and dive into the internal capsule. Subcortically, in the internal capsule, the fibers of the corticospinal tract are consolidated into a much smaller area. A blockage of a small perforating lenticulostriate artery, providing blood supply to the internal capsule, may result in infarction with a fairly equal pattern of weakness involving the opposite face, arm, and leg.

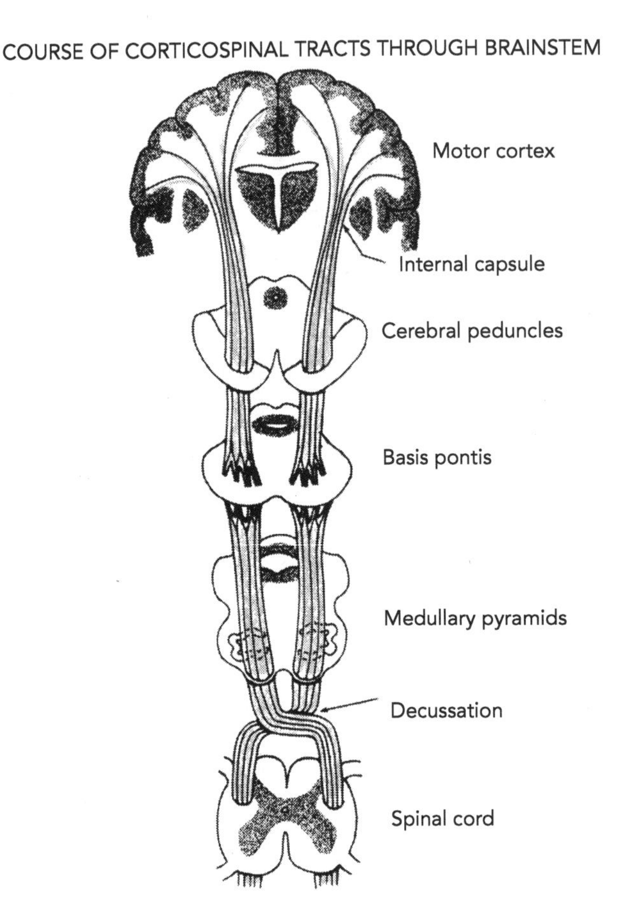

Figure 2.6 The lateral corticospinal tract.

The differential involvement of the face, arm, and leg, as well as attention to involvement of other adjacent structures, is one method of distinguishing a cortical from a subcortical lesion. Tracing lesions down the entire path of a tract or nerve as it winds through the system to reach a target organ or muscle is the beginning of fine tuning the localization process in clinical neurology.

In Figure 2.6, the corticospinal tract crosses in the pyramidal decussation of the inferior ventral medulla. The tract thus ends up on the contralateral side of the spinal cord in the lateral corticospinal tract. If the lesion lies above where this crossover or decussation takes place, the loss seen would be on the contralateral side (i.e., a crossed hemiparesis). There are exceptions of course; for example, a lesion of the ventral medulla at the top of the decussation could affect the crossing upper extremity fibers although sparing the lower extremity ones, leading to a rare cruciate deficit (one where the arms and not the legs are affected). Such findings underscore the importance of anatomy in localization: if it can be understood how the tract functions and travels, a lesion can be localized based on clinical presentation.

Accessory motor area and frontal eye fields

The accessory motor area or premotor cortex (Figure 2.7, Brodmann area 6) is necessary for patterned complex movements. It is here that many commonly used motor sequences are stored, such as the "programs" to run up a flight of stairs or blow out a match. The frontal eye fields (Figure 2.7, Brodmann area 8) are responsible for the initiation of voluntary eye movements. These stimulate conjugate eye movement to the opposite side. For example, the right frontal eye field turns both eyes to the left. A lesion disrupting the right frontal eye field would result in impaired eye movement to the left, or a right gaze preference. That is, the driving force for leftward eye movement is lost. In the subsequent imbalance, the frontal eye fields from the intact left hemisphere take over, and the eyes move toward the right. Conversely, a seizure causing excitation (rather than destruction) of the frontal eye fields will stimulate eye movement toward the opposite side, representing an exaggerated effect by this same cortical region. That is, a right frontal lobe seizure will drive the eyes to the left.

The supplementary motor area (Figure 2.7, Brodmann area 6) controls contraction of the postural muscles. Destruction of this area produces an increase in flexor muscle tone leading to spasmodic contracture and pathological grasp reflexes on both sides. This is a cortical area influencing motor function both contralaterally and ipsilaterally and, hence, represents one of the exceptions to the rule that the brain controls (only) the opposite side of the body.

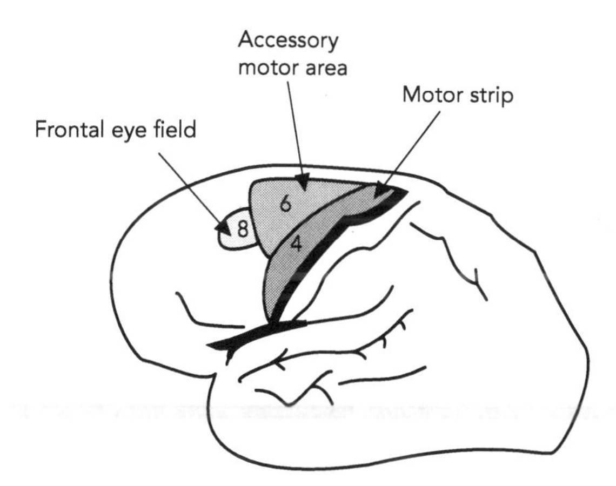

Figure 2.7 The primary motor strip, accessory motor area, and the frontal eye field are all part of the (fabulous) frontal lobe.

Clinicoanatomical correlations of cortical lesions

- Anterior cerebral artery infarction:
  - Weakness of opposite (i.e., contralateral) leg
  - Minimal contralateral arm weakness
  - No facial involvement
  - Normal speech and language

- Middle cerebral artery infarction:
  - Weakness in contralateral face and arm
  - Mild contralateral leg weakness
  - Aphasia (if in the language-dominant hemisphere, which is the left hemisphere for almost all right-handed individuals and about one half of left-handed individuals)
  - Gaze preference toward the lesion

- Frontal lobe tumors:
  - Tumors do not abide by vascular territories. Tumors may recruit extra blood vessels but they do not respect normal vascular boundaries, growing insidiously between connecting pathways and often reaching great size before causing deficits. Their localization is not as *clean* as in the case of vascular strokes.
  - The time course helps to make the diagnosis as much as the localization. Tumors may take time to grow, and the deficits thus tend to progress over time.

- Seizures:

  Seizures originating along the motor strip may produce a Jacksonian march of twitching in the face and limbs in the sequence that they are represented on the motor strip.

> This is named for John Hughlings Jackson, who established the long-standing and dominant neurological unit of The National Hospital, Queen Square, in London, England, during his long tenure there from 1862 until the beginning of the 19th century. Jackson asserted that the nervous system could be viewed as a sensorimotor machine, without a need for reference to metaphysical agents such as the soul. This was a major advance, in contrast to the commonly held physiological viewpoint of his day. His teachings remain influential. His contemporary, Jean-Martin Charcot, at the Salpêtrière Hospital in Paris, France, likewise emphasized clinicoanatomical correlation to study neurological conditions. Allegorically, these men are the fathers of modern neurology.

- Higher executive functions:

  Discussion of the frontal lobes would be incomplete without mentioning that they are the *home* of the higher executive functions, which have varying definitions. Neurologically, the higher executive functions are focusing, concentrating, inhibiting of motor activity, and regulating of sensory input. These processes require coordination among three areas of the prefrontal cortex: the dorsolateral prefrontal cortex (Figure 2.8), the orbitofrontal cortex, and the anterior cingulate gyrus. Together, these areas are required for key functions:

- Planning
- Initiating
- Maintaining
- Self-checking

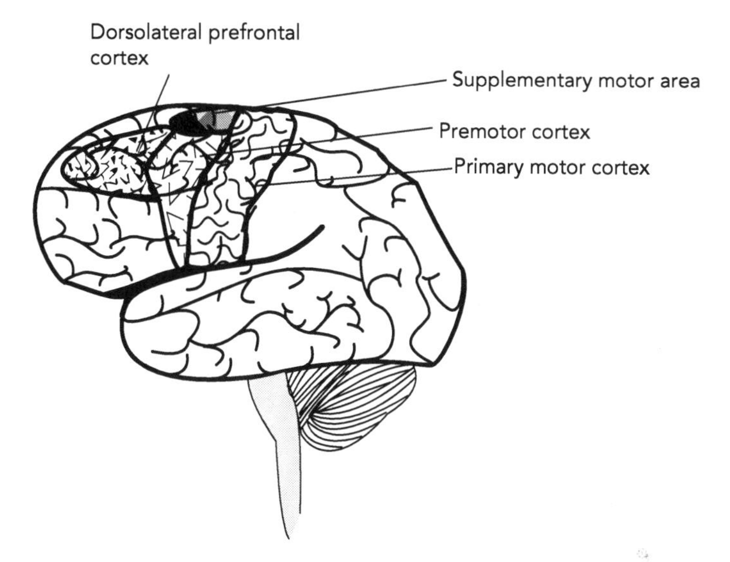

Figure 2.8 Specific frontal lobe regions showing areas devoted to planning and executing of motor activity.

> Think about what it takes to apply to college or medical school. You have to do all the planning and preparatory work; take the right courses in high school and college; and take the entrance examinations. You must initiate the application process, maintain and stick to it, and reevaluate whether it is the right path for you. This all keeps the frontal lobes very active. These aspects are covered more fully in the neuropsychiatry chapter later in this book.

The dorsolateral prefrontal cortex, orbitomedial prefrontal cortex, and anterior cingulate have many connections with limbic structures, particularly the thalamus, the hippocampus, and the amygdala. These cortical–subcortical circuits are involved with the genesis of both normal and abnormal moods, anxiety reactions, and other psychiatric conditions (more details in Chapter 5 on neuropsychiatry).

Fun Fact: The Frontal Lobotomy (So you're considering a career in neurosurgery . . . ?)

- Currently out of vogue.
- Formerly used to control behavior, especially in schizophrenia.
- Results in an intellectually intact individual devoid of emotional responsiveness (slow and apathetic).
- The physiological equivalent occurred to railroad worker Phineas Gage, in whom a penetrating bifrontal injury led to an abulic personality (more details in the neuropsychiatry chapter).

2. Temporal Lobes

The temporal lobe, conveniently located near the temple, lies beneath the Sylvian fissure and extends longitudinally from an anterior pole to its posterior border shared with the occipital and parietal lobes. Its deep structures, although not visible from the outer brain surface, are essential for the properties of memory and emotion, two of the basic characteristics that make us human. The temporal lobe is the site of Wernicke's area, the home of language comprehension, which is linked to Broca's expressive language area of the frontal lobe via the arcuate fasciculus (i.e., an arching subcortical bundle of myelinated fibers) (Figure 2.9). The temporal lobe is also the primary cortical reception area for hearing.

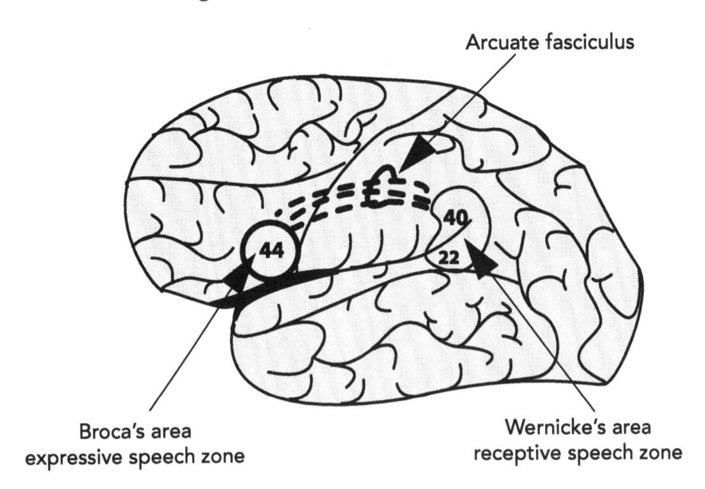

Figure 2.9 Patients with damage to Wernicke's area (Brodmann areas 22 and 40, predominantly superior temporal lobe as well as the junction of where the temporal and parietal lobes meet) will have a receptive aphasia in which they are unable to understand spoken language. This differs from Broca's expressive aphasia in the frontal lobe in which patients are unable to express themselves verbally (Table 2.1).

Summary of temporal lobe functions

- Primary and association (processing) cortex for hearing
- Receptive language
- Memory
- Strong links with the limbic system and emotion

Hearing and auditory processing

The primary auditory cortex corresponds to the transverse gyri of Heschl (Brodmann area 41) and the associative cortex below it (Brodmann area 42). These are two finger-like gyri that lie inside the Sylvian fissure on the superior surface of each temporal lobe (Figure 2.10).

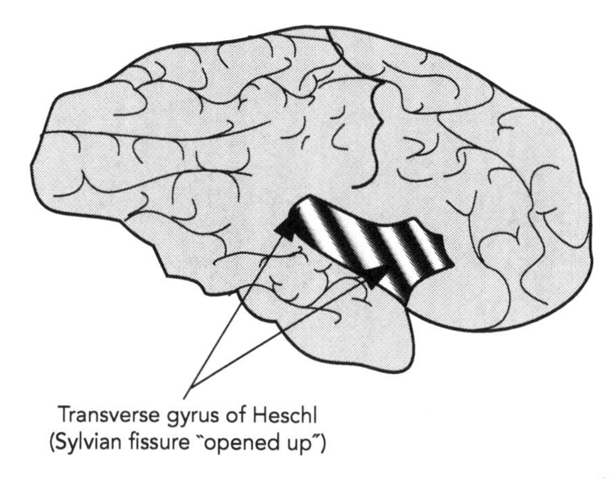

Figure 2.10 The primary auditory cortex is located in the transverse gyri of Heschl (Brodmann area 41) that lies inside the Sylvian fissure on the superior surface of each temporal lobe.

Hearing has bilateral representation in the cerebral cortex, with a stronger contralateral component than in the ipsilateral contribution. Therefore, a unilateral lesion of the auditory cortex produces partial impairment of hearing from the contralateral ear, with a lesser degree of hearing loss from the ipsilateral side. This is often clinically undetectable.

Cortical deafness is extremely rare. It requires bilateral lesions of Heschl's gyri.

Cortical association areas (Brodmann area 42) integrate pure tones into complex sounds with meaning, thereby processing signals that pertain to spoken language. These areas also maintain connections with the entorhinal cortex of the frontal lobe. Disruption of the connections between cortical association areas and the entorhinal cortex may produce anterograde auditory amnesia, in which a patient is unable to retain spoken language. This is an example of the involvement of both auditory processing and memory. It also illustrates the complex processing functions of cortical association areas, as opposed to primary cortical areas such as the precentral motor strip on which the homunculus lives.

Lesions of cortical association areas for hearing result in an inability to recognize familiar sounds as words (dominant hemisphere) or tunes (nondominant hemisphere). This defect is called auditory agnosia. The patient speaks normally but is word deaf (Figure 2.11). The motor correlate of agnosia is apraxia, which means the inability to perform a complex motor task, despite having intact movement and even the ability to perform isolated components but not the whole of the task.

Receptive language

Wernicke's area is located at the posterior temporal lobe, capping the end of the Sylvian fissure and composed of in Brodmann areas 40 and 22 (Figure 2.11). This strategically placed cortical area integrates visual, auditory, and proprioceptive information for the comprehension of language.

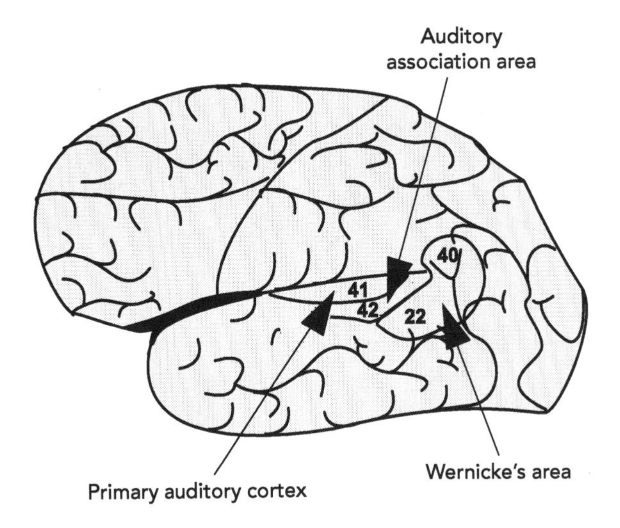

Figure 2.11 The primary auditory cortex (Brodmann area 41) is located just superior to the auditory association area (Brodmann area 42) and is adjacent to Wernicke's area.

Memory and emotion

Memory and emotion are linked, and this complicated human activity is located predominantly in the temporal lobe.

- The hippocampus and dorsomedial nucleus of the thalamus are connected and are important in formation of memories. These structures are part of the limbic system, located near the medial edge of the cerebral cortex (Figure 2.12).
- Bilateral disease of the hippocampus or dorsomedial nucleus of the thalamus results in an inability to form new memories (e.g., Korsakoff psychosis).

- Limbic dysfunction can cause behavioral changes and may underlie a number of psychiatric disorders.

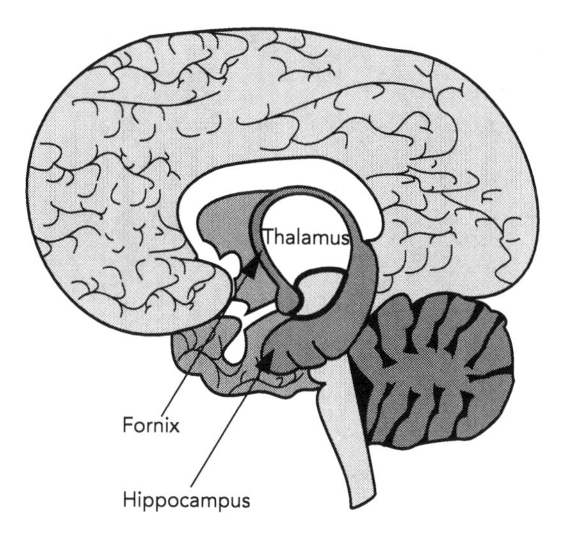

Figure 2.12 The fornix and hippocampus are key components of the limbic system, as are the mediodorsal and anterior nuclei of the thalamus, the amygdala, mammillary bodies, and the hypothalamus.

Focused Highlight on Memory

Memory is complex, and one may initially divide memory into procedural memory for automatic skills (i.e., you never forget how to ride a bike) versus declarative memory for learned information.

Whereas procedural memories are consolidated in the basal ganglia, cerebellum, and frontal lobe (more motorically based areas), declarative memory, at least in a general sense, is predominantly the province of the temporal lobe. In particular, the medial structures (more phylogenetically primitive) help to preserve one's episodic (i.e., autobiographical) memories, and the more temporal neocortical structures (more phylogenetically advanced) help to consolidate the so-called semantic memory, or information-laden material.

Another domain of memory is the evanescent working memory, a higher executive frontal lobe housekeeping function that holds a complex task in your mind long enough to complete it (e.g., remembering how to drive home from work without really thinking about it). A more detailed version of the traditional *Papez circuit,* wherein episodic memories are consolidated by connections among the limbic system, hypothalamus, and thalamus, is shown in Figure 2.13. Figure 2.14 depicts the areas involved in the formation of working, semantic, and procedural memory.

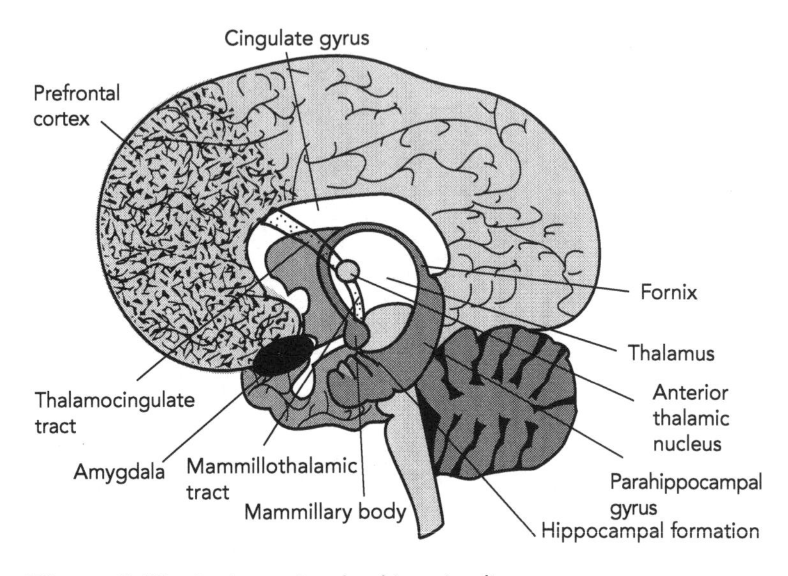

Figure 2.13 Pathways involved in episodic memory.

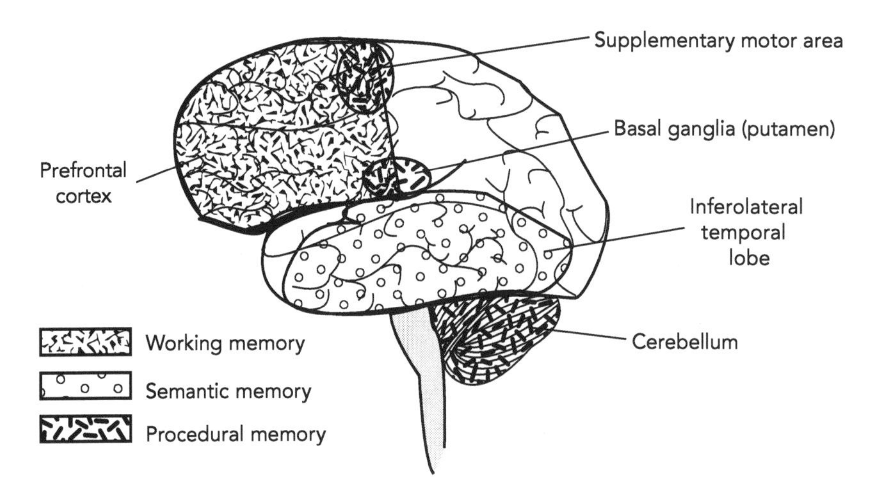

Figure 2.14 Cerebral areas involved in working, semantic, and procedural memory.

Clinicoanatomical correlations

- Korsakoff psychosis etiologies:
  - Heavy chronic alcohol abuse with thiamine deficiency
  - Thiamine deficiency of other etiology (e.g., gastrointestinal disease, malnutrition)
  - Bilateral hippocampal ischemia (Figures 2.15 and 2.16)

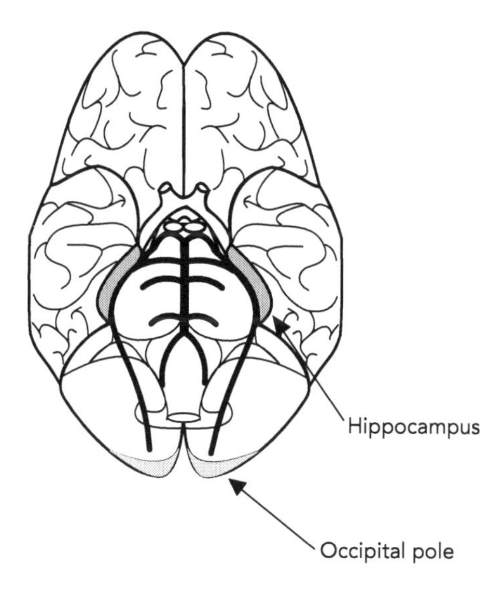

Figure 2.15 The posterior circulation extends to the hippocampi of the deep mesial (medial) temporal lobes and the occipital lobes.

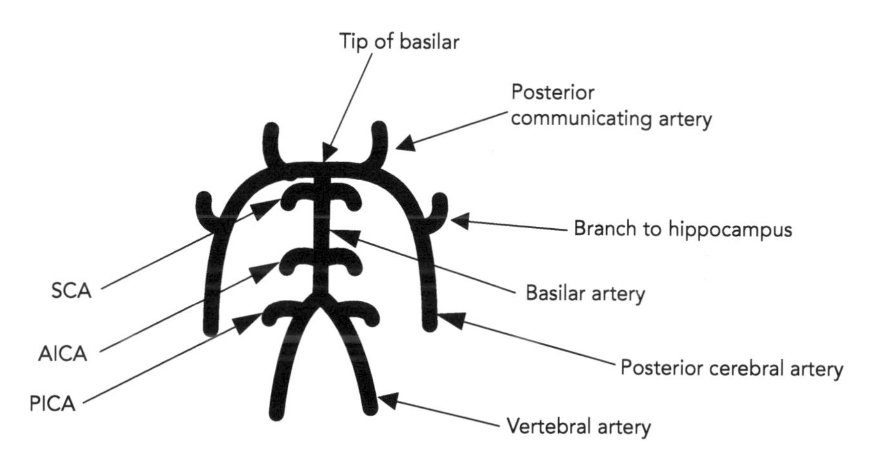

Figure 2.16 Posterior circulation to the brain. Arterial branches of the vertebrobasilar system are shown. The single basilar artery is ultimately responsible for blood flow to much of the brainstem and to both occipital lobes. SCA: Superior cerebellar artery; AICA: Anterior inferior cerebellar artery; PICA: Posterior inferior cerebellar artery.

- Temporal lobe seizures (focal epileptic seizures commonly arise from the limbic structures of the medial temporal lobe). A seizure is an abnormal electrical discharge from neurons. Seizures may emanate in particular from the limbic structures of the medial temporal lobe. Characteristics of medial temporal lobe seizures include:
  - Hallucinations: olfactory, auditory, or formed visual images. The temporal lobe has connections to the entorhinal cortex, leading to

the connection to the olfactory system. Auditory hallucinations may represent primary psychiatric disease but also may be seen in temporal lobe epilepsy, attributable to epileptic activation of the auditory cortex. Although the primary visual cortex is located in the occipital lobe, temporal lobe association cortex acts to process and integrate multimodal sensory information, so that formed, complex visual imagery (i.e., seeing faces or animals as opposed to simple flashes of light or patterns) may occur due to temporal lobe seizures.

- Complex movements: these are often stereotypical movements, known as automatisms, done in a state of clouded consciousness. Think of the unnatural movements of a robot or automaton. A perseverative automatism would indicate ongoing, albeit altered, movements that were already in place at the onset of a seizure (e.g., a person dealing a deck of cards may continue but in a nonfluid way). This is in contrast to a de novo automatism, where people would start licking their lips, smacking their lips, or pulling at their clothes in the middle of a seizure.
- Fugue-like states: these are long states of altered consciousness where individuals are found in a trance and unaware of their surroundings yet, unwittingly, could have traveled for miles.
- Deja vu/jamais vu: here the temporal lobe is really playing tricks with one's mind, with the feeling that something unique had happened in the same way before, or that something that had happened before was now unique, respectively.

The aphasias! Putting the frontal and temporal lobes together

Aphasia is a disturbance of language function that resides in the dominant hemisphere. The left hemisphere is dominant for language in practically all right-handed individuals as well as the majority (nearly 80%, according to fMRI [functional magnetic resonance imaging] language studies) of left-handed persons. (Many left-handed people claim that only they are in their "right minds." You may choose to believe them, but in truth, only a minority are right-brain dominant.)

Language representation in the brain may be divided into two main areas: the frontal lobe just anterior to the lip region of the homunculus (Broca's area for expressive language) and the temporal lobe (Wernicke's area for receptive language) (Figure 2.9). This follows the scheme that frontal lobe functioning is centered on motor activity because a frontal lobe aphasia will principally involve the motoric (i.e., expressive) aspects of language. Therefore, the patient with Broca's aphasia is not fluent, yet will retain comprehension of language. In contrast, a Wernicke's aphasia is a sensory or receptive aphasia, where speech is fluent and language may consist of nonsensical *word salad* but language comprehension is missing.

In Wernicke's area, the processing of visual, auditory, and proprioceptive inputs leads to assignment of a vocabulary and syntax. This receptive area is connected to Broca's motor area via the *arcuate fasciculus*, thus allowing for word concepts to be transformed into verbal speech output.

- Types of aphasia:
  - Expressive aphasia (synonyms: Broca's aphasia, motor aphasia, nonfluent aphasia, anterior aphasia)
    - Fluency—decreased; speech is hesitant and may be low in volume or absent
    - Content—appropriate; overly semantic without connector words; fragments of nouns produced can often be pieced together to make sense
    - Frustration—a great deal of effort is expended attempting to verbalize
    - Comprehension—intact
    - Repetition—impaired
    - Naming—variably affected, at times with paraphasic errors of the phonemic type (i.e., the patient responds "pam" when asked to name a pen).

Example: The patient watched a video clip of a dog fetching a ball, knocking over a toddler, and then stopping to lick the child. The patient was asked to describe what happened and said, "Dog...running...ball... fall down...ah, it is wet."

  - Receptive aphasia (synonyms: Wernicke's aphasia, sensory aphasia, fluent aphasia, posterior aphasia)
    - Fluency—normal; volume may be increased
    - Content—despite intact speech fluency, the language is devoid of meaning; words themselves are often malformed or jargon, bearing no relation to real words (neologisms)
    - Complacency—the effortful frustration in the expressive aphasias is not evident
    - Comprehension—severely disturbed
    - Repetition—variably affected
    - Naming—impaired with paraphasic errors of the semantic type (wrong meaning) and neologisms

Example: The patient was shown the same video described above and asked to describe the scene. He had trouble understanding what was requested and said, "I am high low running over the hills borgly basket toys going home."

These are the classical aphasias. Other aphasias produce variations on these themes. Recall that the arcuate fasciculus (an *arc* for arcuate, and *fasciculus* for track of myelinated axons) joins the temporal, receptive language area of Wernicke to the frontal, expressive language region of Broca. Lesions of this tract cause conduction aphasia, marked by an inability to repeat. There are transcortical motor and sensory aphasias, secondary to brain lesions in the cortex surrounding Broca's and Wernicke's areas, respectively. These aphasias have the characteristics of the motor and sensory aphasias, except with preserved ability to repeat.

Anomia is a relatively nonlocalizing finding, and anomic aphasia is characterized by primary inability to name objects. Large lesions (e.g., strokes or tumors) may produce global aphasia, which is a combination of expressive and receptive aphasia. Even lesions of subcortical structures, such as the thalamus, can be associated with aphasias. In thalamic aphasia, repetition is spared, and there is usually more rapid recovery than with the cortical aphasias. The cardinal features of the various aphasias are shown in Table 2.1.

The cerebral aphasias should not be confused with communication dysfunction that can occur in other conditions—for example, cerebellar mutism following posterior fossa surgery (especially removal of a cerebellar tumor), hypoglossal or vagus nerve damage (changes in speech tone), or disarticulation related to oromotor coordination. In addition, it may be challenging to distinguish the impaired awareness of encephalopathic processes causing confusion and disorientation from impaired language of dysphasia.

Some aphasias, particularly Broca's, may be associated with articulatory difficulty and slurred speech (dysarthria). Problems with articulation may also be seen in the absence of language dysfunction, in patients with lesions affecting the brainstem cranial nerve nuclei innervating the muscles of the tongue and articulation.

Table 2.1 Cardinal Features of the Various Aphasias

Type of aphasia	Fluency	Comprehension	Repetition	Naming
Broca's	–	+	–	–
Transcortical motor	–	+	+	–
Wernicke's	+	–	–	–
Transcortical sensory	+	–	+	–
Conduction	+	+	–	–
Global	–	–	–	–
Anomic	+	+	+	–
Thalamic	+/–	+/–	+	–

Note: +, retained; –, lost.

3. Parietal Lobes

The parietal lobe begins with the postcentral gyrus, just behind the Sylvian fissure, and extends posteriorly to the anterior margin of the occipital lobe and inferiorly to the Sylvian fissure overlying the temporal lobe (Figure 2.17). The postcentral gyrus is the parietal primary sensory strip, and is somatotopically organized with the sensory homunculus, analogous to the motor strip (Figure 2.18). This homunculus is formed according to the innervation density of the body part. Again, note the vast representation of the face, tongue, and hand.

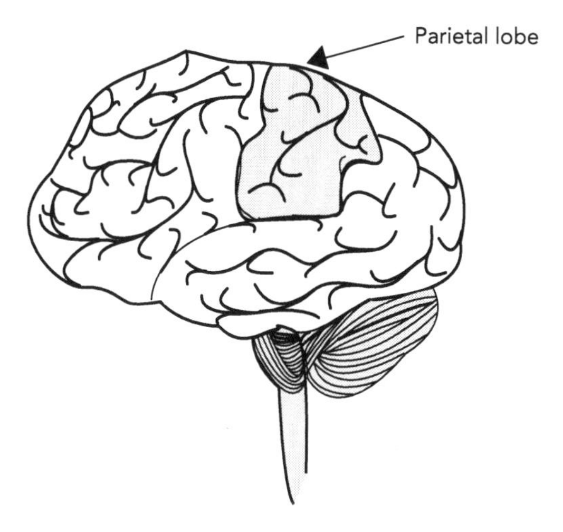

Figure 2.17 The parietal lobe extends posteriorly from the central sulcus to the parieto-occipital boundary.

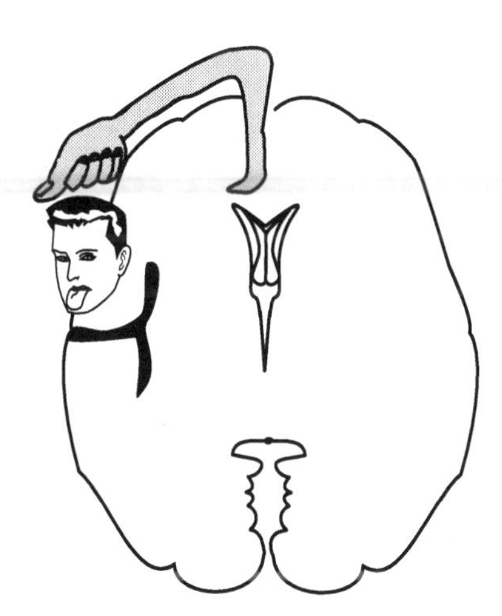

Figure 2.18 The sensory version of the homunculus: HAL (head, arm, leg).

The remainder of the parietal lobe is a sensory integrating center. The confluence of incoming sensory information is integrated in the parietal lobe to produce an ongoing awareness of corporeal and extracorporeal space. Think of the parietal lobe as having a screen with a continually updated image of the body in space. With intact parietal lobe function, individuals can close their eyes, stretch out one arm with thumb up, and grab the thumb with the other hand. Parietal lobe functioning is clinically assessed during the sensory part of the neurological examination. Although the primary sensory modalities such as light touch, sharp touch, temperature, and proprioception (joint position sense) are registered at the spinal cord and thalamic levels, the secondary, or higher cortical, sensory modalities are the province of the parietal lobe. These are the ability to perceive more complicated sensory input: graphesthesia (e.g., palm writing), stereognosia (interpreting objects by shape), two-point discrimination (discernment of discrete simultaneous stimuli at close distances), complex proprioception (perception of complex body movements and postures in three-dimensional space), and comparative weights (differentiating a heavier from a lighter object).

Extinction occurs when, despite having the sensory ability to discern a stimulus presented to either side of the body, a patient fails to recognize the stimulus on one side when presented with bilateral or double simultaneous stimulation (Figure 2.19).

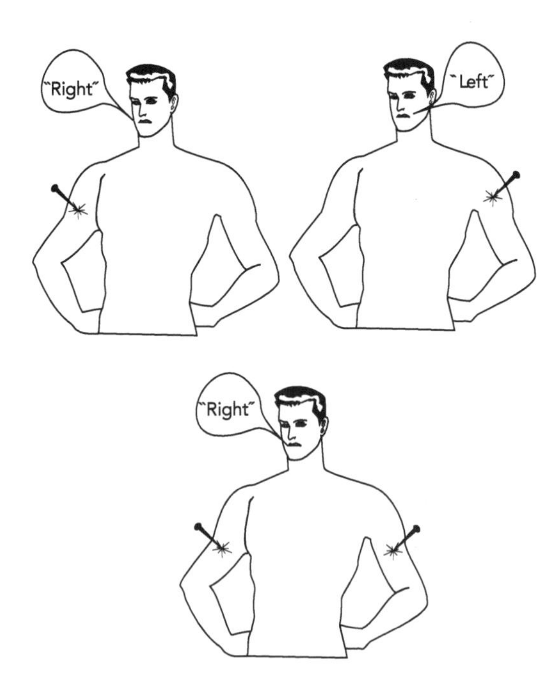

Figure 2.19 Presentation of extinction. "Bob" may be able to feel a stimulus on the right or left side separately but when presented with double simultaneous stimuli, he fails to discern the left-sided stimulus.

Dominant and nondominant (neglect) parietal syndromes

A related and peculiar feature of parietal lobe pathology is that of spatial neglect. That is, the parietal lobe is instrumental in our ability to attend to our environment. In the case of spatial comprehension, the parietal lobe in the nondominant hemisphere is dominant. The nondominant (right—most often the case) parietal lobe actually pays attention to both sides of space, whereas the dominant (left) attends to only the contralateral side. Therefore, a dominant (left) parietal lobe lesion does not lead to right-sided neglect because the nondominant (right) parietal lobe takes over, attending to both sides of space. In a nondominant (right) parietal lesion, however, there is no reserve system to attend to the left side of space. Hence, we see hemineglect syndromes on the left in the event of right parietal lobe lesions.

What does it mean to neglect one side of space? It can mean that a patient eats from only the right side of the tray, or neglects to shave the left side of the face, or fails to draw in the left side of the clock face from 6:00 to 12:00. It may lead to the alien hand syndrome, where the patient interprets one's own left hand as belonging to a stranger.

- Clinical findings in parietal lobe syndromes:
  - Agraphesthesia—letters or numbers written on the palm of the hand are not recognized.
  - Astereognosis—objects placed in the palm of the hand are not recognized.
  - Loss of two-point tactile discrimination—as stimuli are presented closer and closer, there is loss of appreciation of two discrete stimuli.
  - Extinction—sensory stimuli are presented bilaterally and simultaneously, yet not perceived on the side opposite a parietal lesion.

- Classical findings associated with nondominant parietal lobe lesions:
  - Asomatognosia—inability to recognize one's own body parts on the affected side and to localize them in space.
  - Dressing apraxia—inability to properly arrange clothing on oneself.
  - Constructional apraxia—inability to draw or copy diagrams.
  - Geographic disorientation—inability to form a conceptual map of an area.

- Classical findings associated with dominant parietal lobe lesions:

  The Gerstmann syndrome is a tetrad of deficits associated with dominant parietal lobe lesions.

  - Right–left confusion—the patient can no longer recognize left versus right.
  - Finger agnosia—the patient is not able to name or differentiate the fingers.
  - Acalculia—loss of arithmetic skills.
  - Agraphia—loss of writing skills.

Note: Dementias with prominent involvement of the parietal lobe may present with disorientation in extracorporeal space (i.e., Grandma gets lost driving home from the grocery store).

Optokinetic nystagmus

Notice that in a moving car or train, a passenger's eyes fixate and refixate while traveling past trees, signs, or people. This is a normal physiological type of nystagmus known as optokinetic nystagmus (OKN). It is also helpful in parietal lobe testing.

OKN may be elicited by moving a striped tape across the visual field (Figure 2.20). The eyes follow the stimulus briefly and then return in a rapid jerky movement to the midline. In a patient with a parietal lobe lesion, the response is absent when the strip is moved toward the abnormal parietal lobe.

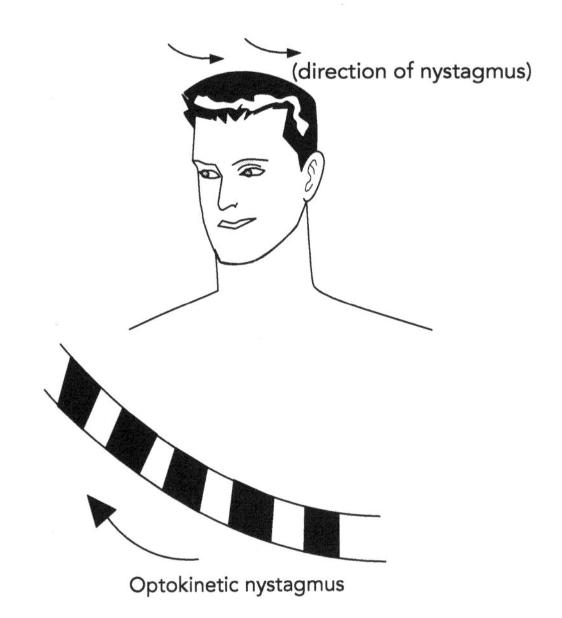

Figure 2.20 Optokinetic nystagmus (OKN) is a normal reflexive eye movement allowing for refixation to moving visual stimuli. The patient should demonstrate the normal pursuit movement and then refixation nystagmus when a striped tape is moved from left to right. If OKNs are absent, a right hemispheric (typically parietal) lesion is suggested.

4. Occipital Lobes

The occipital lobe is at the back of the brain, demarcated by the parieto-occipital sulcus superiorly and the calcarine sulcus inferiorly (Figure 2.21). The primary visual cortex is the calcarine cortex (Brodmann area 17). This is the principal area for visual perception, integration, and formation of binocular images. Directly in front are the visual association cortices, Brodmann areas 18 and 19 (Figure 2.22). Whereas the afferent visual pathways terminate here, consideration of the visual field defects requires review of the entire length of the pathway.

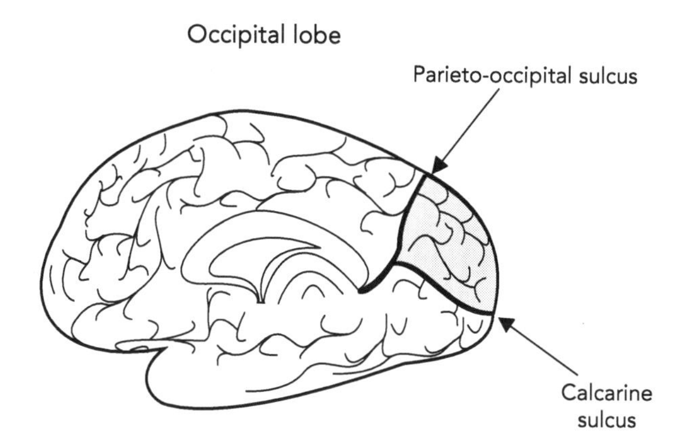

Figure 2.21 The parieto-occipital sulcus marks the superior border of the occipital lobe, whereas the calcarine sulcus demarcates the inferior border.

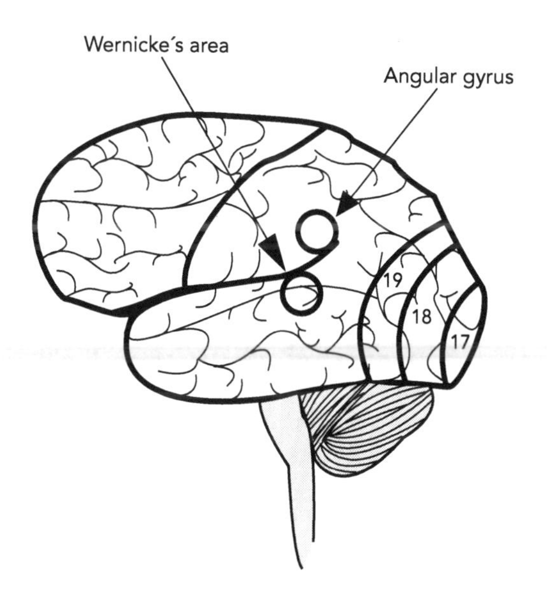

Figure 2.22 Calcarine cortex (primary visual cortex, Brodmann area 17) is shown along with the visual association cortices (Brodmann areas 18 and 19). Lesions of the dominant angular gyrus lead to disruption of sensory association cortex and Gerstmann syndrome, the tetrad of dysgraphia, acalculia, left–right confusion, and finger agnosia.

Occipital lobe function

Examination of the patient's visual fields is a method to assess occipital lobe function as well as the earlier, more proximal, portions of the visual pathway. The discrete organization of the visual field information in the visual pathways allows visual field assessment, to provide accurate lesion localization. Visual fields can be tested at the bedside by using confrontation testing. The examiner should test each eye separately by covering one eye at a time. It is also essential to test each quadrant while watching the patient carefully for central fixation. Asking the patient to count the number of fingers presented in each visual quadrant is usually the optimal method at the bedside. Moving or wiggling fingers may be needed to test some patients, especially children; however, this technique is less sensitive than finger counting for detecting regions of mildly decreased vision. A red match or similar object also enhances the sensitivity of the test because red desaturation is a subtle and early sign of optic neuropathy. At some point during the examination the fingers should be held up simultaneously on the right and left sides to test for extinction, a sign of visual neglect. Conventionally, visual fields are recorded with the right eye on the right side of the page—as if viewing one's own visual field. In the case of a patient in whom it is unclear whether there is any vision, testing for "blink to threat" by approaching the patient with a rapid flicker of the hand can be a useful way of grossly testing visual fields.

More formal visual field testing is done by presenting objects throughout the central and peripheral visual fields utilizing a technique known as perimetry, either manually (Goldmann perimetry) or automatically (computerized perimetry). Figure 2.23 shows the visual field defects expected in the case of a lesion at different locations in the optic pathway. This pathway begins with the eye, of course, and the optic nerve is discussed later with the cranial nerves. But an overview of the visual pathway is helpful at this point.

The visual pathway begins with the retina. When visual images initially activate the photoreceptors (i.e., rods and cones) in the deepest layer of the retina, an electrical signal is transmitted proximally until reaching the axons of the outermost layer, which form the optic nerve (cranial nerve II). As light enters the eye and passes through the lens onto the retina, images are both reversed and inverted. The nasal half of the retina sees the temporal half of the environment, and the temporal half of the retina sees the nasal portion of the environment. Closing one eye, note that the temporal visual field of one eye is larger than the nasal portion. The optic nerves cross at the optic chiasm, and here the nasal fibers from one eye decussate to join the temporal fibers from the other eye. Hence, the left hemisphere beyond the optic chiasm sees the nasal half of space from the left eye, and the temporal part of space from the right eye (i.e., the right side of space). This is yet another example of one cerebral hemisphere being concerned with the opposite side of space. Whereas a lesion of one optic nerve will interfere with vision from only that eye, a lesion in the body of the optic chiasm will preferentially involve the crossing nasal retinal fibers, and hence impair vision from each temporal, or lateral, side of space. This is known as a bitemporal hemianopia.

Following their decussation in the optic chiasm, the optic nerves then become the optic tracts that synapse onto the lateral geniculate nucleus of the thalamus. The postsynaptic fibers then travel through the subcortical white matter and fan out as the optic radiations; superior fibers traversing the parietal lobe see the lower half of the visual field, and inferior fibers traversing down through the temporal lobe see the upper half of the visual field. The theme of light being reversed and inverted as it enters the eye is consistent throughout the pathway.

The optic radiations join together as they enter the occipital lobe, where they synapse onto the calcarine cortex. There are several principles of visual fields that help to localize defects to the occipital lobe versus more proximal brain regions. As fibers reach their final destination, they join each other in tighter bundles rather than being fanned out. Lesions are more likely to affect the fibers equally, hence leading to a more even field defect. That is, defects are more likely to be the same or congruous. Thus, the more similarly a visual field defect affects both eyes, the more likely it is explained by an abnormality involving the contralateral occipital lobe (as opposed to optic radiations in the parietal or temporal lobe). In addition, fibers serving the central vision of the macula come together tightly and synapse at their own site at the very innermost folding of the calcarine gyrus. The central vision (i.e., macular) fibers are very numerous and tend to be affected in lesions along the pathways of the optic tracts and radiations. Yet the closer to their calcarine home, the more likely the macular fibers will be spared if there is an occipital lobe lesion. An additional reason is this cortical area has a dual blood supply, corresponding to a watershed zone supplied by both the posterior cerebral artery and posterior branches of the middle cerebral artery. Hence, a lesion of one vascular territory will lead to a visual field defect corresponding to the opposite visual field (contralateral hemianopia) but will lead to sparing of the macular fibers and thus preservation of the contralateral half of central vision (i.e., macular sparing). In conclusion, both a congruous homonymous defect and macular sparing support a more occipital than parietal or temporal localization. A summary of visual field defects based on the localization of lesions follows.

Rules of visual field defects (Figure 2.23)

A Optic nerve lesions (prechiasmal) affect one eye and tend to include a central scotoma (blind spot).
B Chiasmal lesions are associated with bitemporal hemianopia.
C Retrochiasmal lesions cause contralateral hemianopias and involve the optic tracts, optic radiations, or occipital lobe(s).
D Parietal lobe lesions cause contralateral inferior quadrantanopias.
E Temporal lobe lesions cause contralateral superior quadrantanopias.

F Occipital lobe lesions cause contralateral hemianopias or quadrantanopias when more limited:
- Lesions to the upper bank of the calcarine fissure: contralateral inferior quadrantanopia
- Lesions to the lower bank of the calcarine fissure: contralateral superior quadrantanopia

---

Note: The more congruous the defect, the more occipital the lesion. The more macular-sparing, the more occipital the lesion.

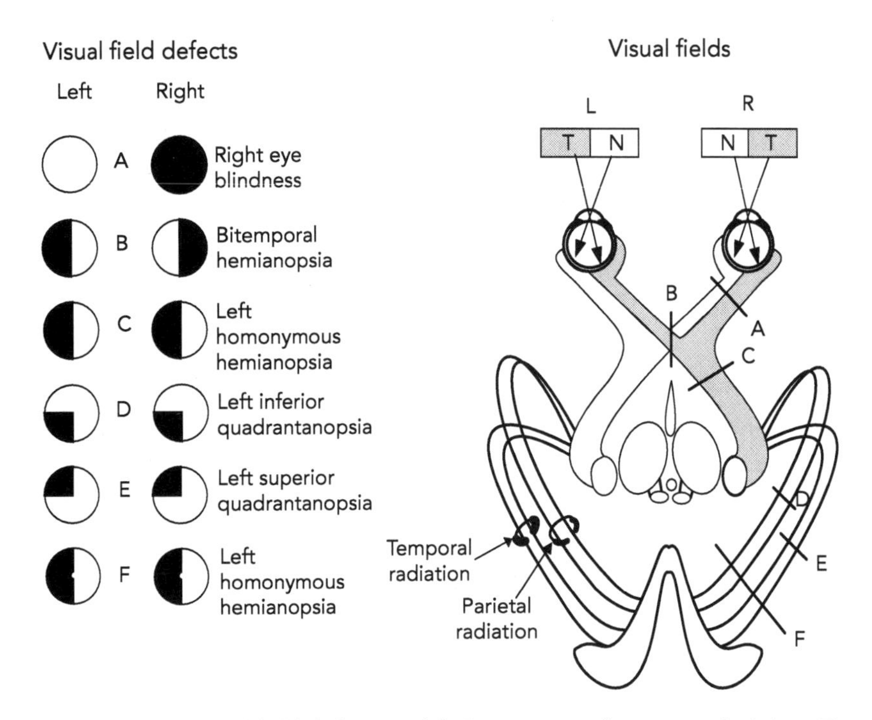

Figure 2.23 Visual field defects and their corresponding anatomical sites. The left panel shows the pictorial demonstration of visual field defects and indicates what the patient sees. The right panel shows the corresponding site of the lesion producing the same defect as indicated by the letters A–F.

Clinicoanatomical correlates of the occipital lobe

- Disconnection syndrome:

  Lesions affecting the left visual cortex and corpus callosum isolate the functional right occipital cortex from the language areas of the left hemisphere. That is, visual information entering the right occipital lobe cannot be transmitted over to the language areas. Affected patients cannot read, yet can write (alexia without agraphia; Figure 2.24).

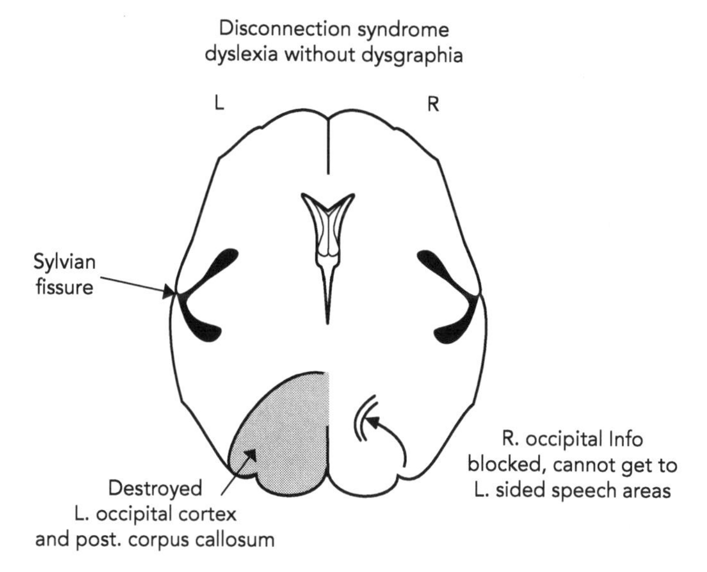

Figure 2.24 Lesions affecting the left visual cortex and corpus callosum prevent transmission of visual information from the right occipital lobe to the left-sided language areas.

- Cortical blindness:

  Lesions of both occipital poles result in loss of cortical areas for sight despite normal eyes. Oddly, patients may deny their blindness (Anton syndrome) confabulating that they can see when obviously they cannot. Etiologies include:

  - Blood clot at the tip of the basilar artery causing ischemia of both posterior cerebral arteries
  - Infarction of one occipital lobe, followed later by infarction of the other
  - Tumor of falx cerebri sitting between occipital poles (Figure 2.25)
  - Prolonged hypotension (postcardiac arrest)
  - Basilar artery migraine

The phenomenon of confabulation is fascinating. In the absence of incoming sensory information the brain tends to fill in the blanks and provide information, even if incorrect. In Anton syndrome, the patient may stumble about the room, clearly visually impaired. Yet, when asked, the patient does not admit or recognize the blindness. If fingers are held up and the number queried, the patient will simply make up an answer. This intriguing syndrome is usually seen only transiently after a bilateral occipital lobe insult.

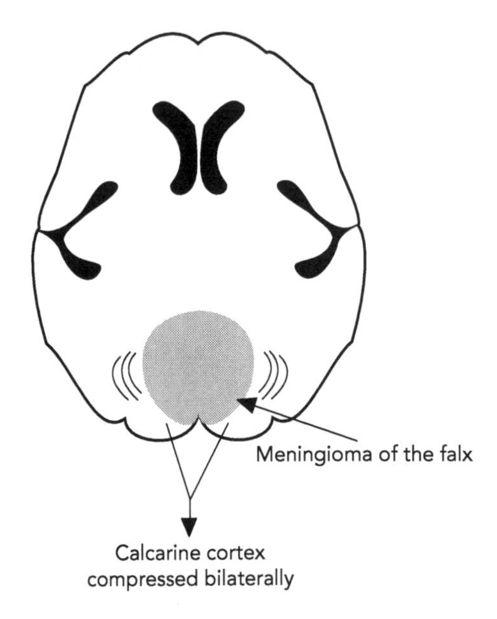

Figure 2.25 A tumor of the falx cerebri sitting between the occipital poles can compress the calcarine cortex causing cortical blindness.

- Occipital seizures:

  Seizures involving the occipital lobe may present with unformed visual hallucinations (i.e., visualization of bright lights [phosphenes], zigzag patterns, or blind spots [scotomata]). This is in contrast to more anterior irritation involving the angular gyrus or temporal lobe that may be associated with more complex visual phenomena (e.g., seeing animals or human faces).

B. THE CRANIAL NERVES AND BRAINSTEM: TRULY VITAL STUFF

The brainstem is organized from top to bottom into three sections: midbrain, pons, and medulla (Figure 2.26).

An overview of the cranial nerves as they exit the ventral brainstem is shown in Figure 2.27.

1. Olfactory Nerve—CN I

Anatomy (Figure 2.21)

- There are chemoreceptor cells in the mucous membrane of the nasal cavity.
- Axons of the chemoreceptor cells pass through the cribriform plate of the ethmoid bone and join together in the olfactory bulbs (Figure 2.28).

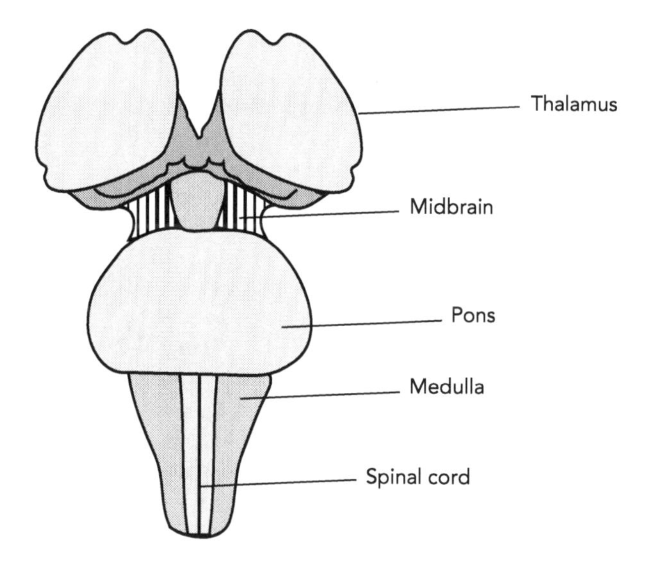

Figure 2.26 Overall organization of the brainstem.

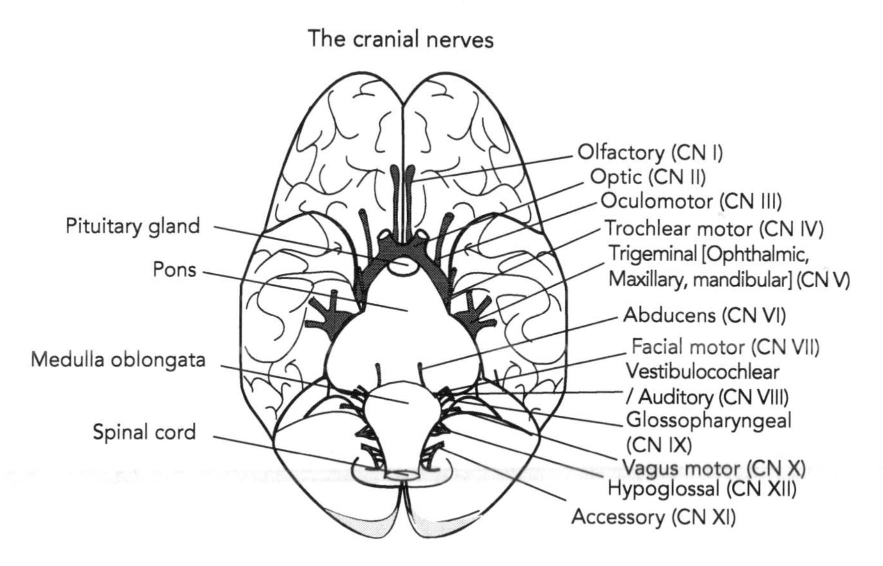

Figure 2.27 Exiting cranial nerves from the ventral brainstem.

- These become the olfactory tracts that carry information to olfactory processing areas including the piriform cortex, amygdala, and entorhinal cortex. These areas project to the thalamus, frontal cortex, and hippocampus (Figure 2.29). The connections form the basis of the intimate association between smell and emotion. Olfaction is the one sensory modality that does not have to pass through the thalamus before cortical processing.

> Fun Fact
> Humans have approximately 5 cm of olfactory epithelium folded within the nose.

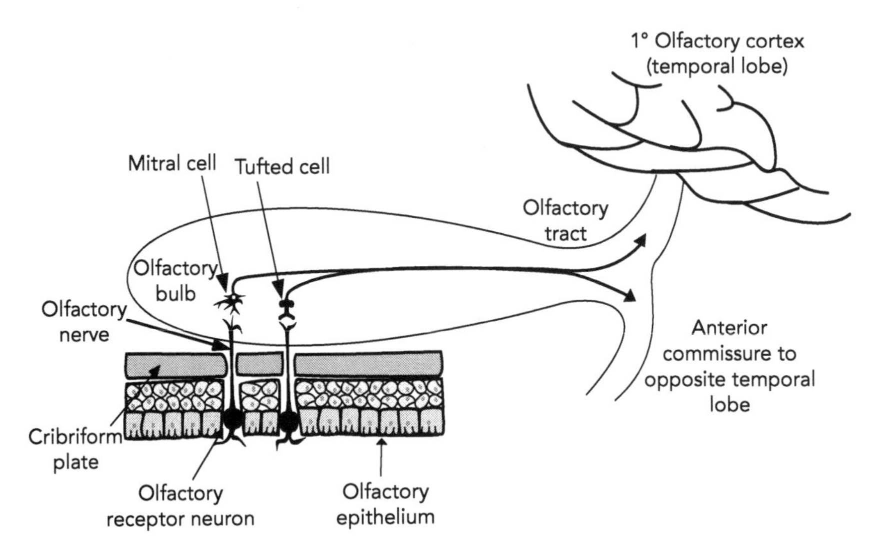

Figure 2.28 Axons of olfactory receptor neurons join to form the bulb and tract of the olfactory nerves that project to the olfactory processing areas and their connections.

Pathology

- The cardinal feature of olfactory nerve dysfunction is anosmia. Note that it is important to examine each nostril separately. Olfactory loss is often not noticed by the patient if it is unilateral because the contralateral nostril is able to compensate. Unilateral anosmia is almost always due to local nasal or sinus disease. Bilateral anosmia raises concern about a neurological lesion, such as an olfactory groove mass in the base of the frontal cranial fossa (e.g., meningioma) or a developmental problem of the rhombencephalon (e.g., Kallman syndrome, an x-linked syndrome of hypothalamic hypogonadism and anosmia).

- Etiologies of anosmia:
    - Heavy smoking
    - Chronic rhinitis
    - Influenza
    - Head injury

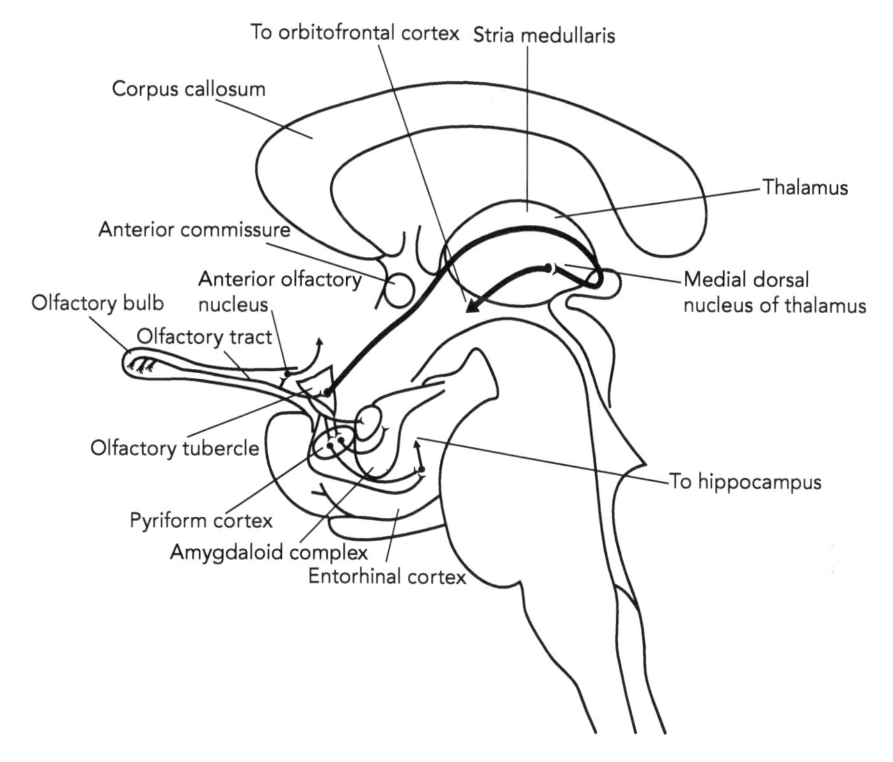

Figure 2.29 Projections of the olfactory pathway.

- Subarachnoid hemorrhage
- Tumor at base of frontal skull
- Meningitis

2. Optic Nerve—CN II

Anatomy

The optic nerve is a direct extension of CNS white matter, and can be viewed directly by identifying the optic disc during funduscopic examination. The optic nerve is assessed clinically by several modalities:

- Pupillary responses to light. The optic nerve represents the afferent end of this reflex arc. (The efferent end is CN III, the oculomotor nerve, discussed later.)
- Visual acuity. This may be done with a card at near vision (e.g., Snellen card) or with a wall chart placed 20 feet in front of the patient.
- Visual fields (discussed in the earlier section regarding the occipital lobe).

- Funduscopy
- Color vision. Loss of red perception occurs early with optic nerve lesions.
- Visual evoked response (VER). Presentation of an alternating checkerboard image with electrical recording of summated and averaged evoked potentials over the occipital cortex—mapping and measuring the signal as it travels from the retina through the lateral geniculate bodies of the thalamus—along the optic radiations to the occipital lobes. The latency of the main waveform, known as the P100 (positive wave at approximately 100 milliseconds), is exquisitely sensitive to demyelinating lesions of the optic nerves.

Pathology

- Optic neuritis. Refers to inflammation of the optic nerve. It may be seen as a parainfectious disorder related to inflammation incited by an immunological response to (typically viral) infection or related to demyelination as in multiple sclerosis.
- Relative afferent pupillary defect (RAPD). The Marcus Gunn Pupil (named for Dr. Robert Marcus Gunn, 1850–1909). A RAPD is a sign of an optic neuropathy. The RAPD is detected utilizing the swinging flashlight test. A pen light is shined in one eye, which should normally lead to constriction of that eye (direct response) and the other eye (consensual response). When the light is then swung to the other eye, that eye should remain constricted if the direct response is intact. If there is a RAPD, that eye will dilate from the previously constricted position relative to the other eye. This dilated eye has impairment of the afferent (not efferent, or CN III) loop of the pupillary light reflex. This is the so-called APD or Marcus Gunn Pupil.

> The term "afferent" refers to incoming sensory information; "efferent" refers to outgoing motor responses.

3. Oculomotor Nerve—CN III

Anatomy (Figure 2.30)

- Nucleus is located in the midbrain.
- CN III exits the brainstem ventrally in the interpeduncular fossa, traverses the cavernous sinus along with CN IV and VI, and then exits the skull via the superior orbital fissure.
- Innervates levator palpebrae superioris as well as all extraocular muscles except the lateral rectus (CN VI) and superior oblique (CN IV) muscles.

- Carries fibers from the Edinger-Westphal nucleus (parasympathetic) to pupilloconstrictor muscle and to the ciliary muscle for accommodation. These parasympathetic fibers are wrapped delicately around the outside of the main CN III nerve trunk and may be impaired by external compression leading to pupillary dilatation (Figure 2.31).
- One of three nerves to the extraocular muscles. The other two are CN IV and CN VI.

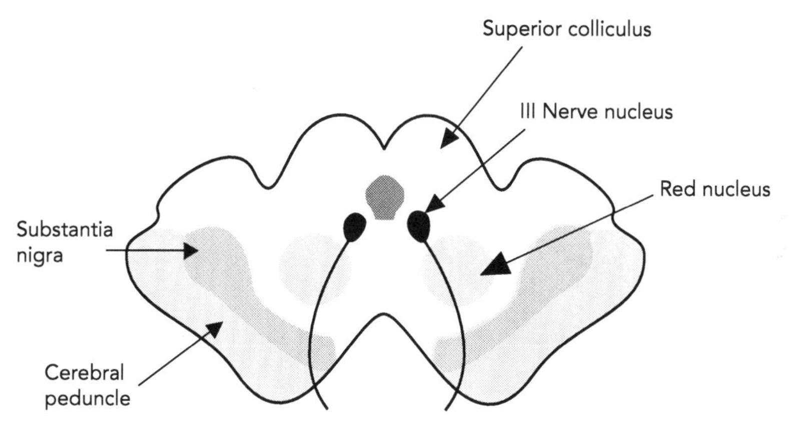

Figure 2.30 Cross-section of midbrain showing course of the exiting oculomotor nerves.

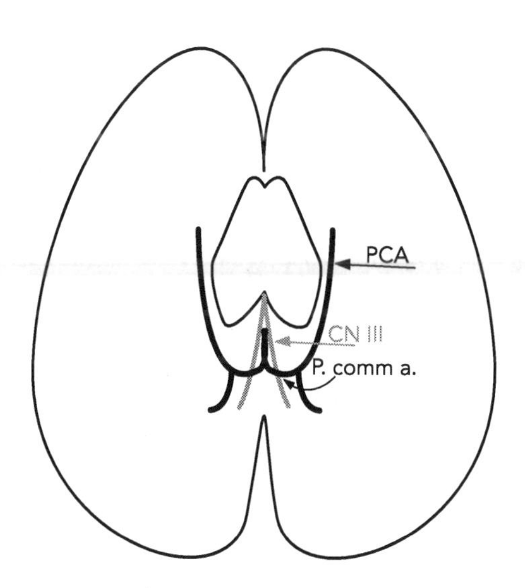

Figure 2.31 Aneurysms of the posterior communicating artery may compress CN III, causing an oculomotor palsy that dilates the pupil due to interference with the superficial parasympathetic pupilloconstrictor fibers.

Pathology

- Midbrain
  - Infarction and tumors may affect CN III in the midbrain.
  - Associated long tract and cerebellar signs help localize the lesion.

- Along base of brain

  CN III passes under the posterior communicating artery. Aneurysms of the posterior communicator may press on CN III. External pressure disturbs the outermost fibers of the nerve that are parasympathetic pupilloconstrictors (Figure 2.32).

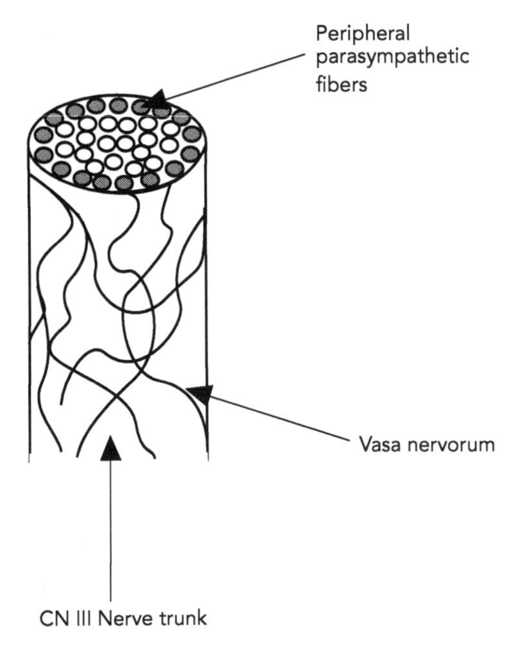

Figure 2.32 Nerve fibers of CN III that innervate the extraocular muscle (EOM) fibers are distributed throughout the nerve trunk, whereas parasympathetic pupilloconstrictor nerve fibers are distributed around the external perimeter. An intrinsic or noncompressive lesion of CN III will affect EOMs but spare the pupils. A compressive lesion, however, will more likely lead to pupillary dilation due to interference with the external pupilloconstrictor fibers.

Disruption of the pupilloconstrictor fibers leaves unopposed sympathetic pupillodilatory action on the pupil, which is normally maintained by balanced constrictor and dilatory influences. Therefore, pupillary dilatation is an early sign of a compressive CN III lesion. Aneurysms typically cause a painful oculomotor palsy that dilates the pupil. The oculomotor palsy may be subtle or complete.

Clinical setting: A 40-year-old man with sudden onset of severe headache comes to the emergency room (ER). Examination is normal except for a poorly reactive right pupil of 5 mm diameter (versus a normal 3 mm and reactive left pupil). This could be a sign of an aneurysm of the right posterior communicating artery.

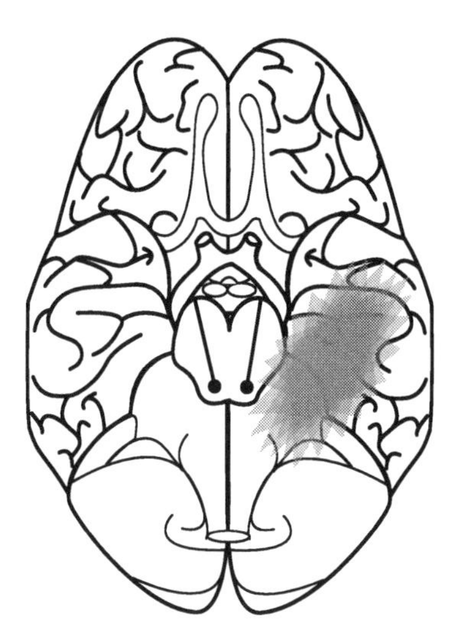

Figure 2.33 Uncal herniation can also compress CN III causing a dilated or "blown" pupil.

In the same region, the nerve passes adjacent to the medial temporal lobe, a region known as the uncus. An enlarging temporal lobe lesion such as a hemorrhage may rapidly reach a critical volume and mass effect. This may lead to a bulging of the medial portion of the uncus over the edge of the falx cerebri, resulting in external compression of CN III (Figure 2.33). In this condition, known as uncal herniation, there is a dilated pupil due to interference with the external pupilloconstrictor fibers. In addition to an ipsilateral CN III palsy, uncal herniation can also result in coma due to brainstem compression.

The motor deficits in uncal herniation would be expected to be contralateral due to direct involvement of the internal capsule and descending corticospinal track on the side of the lesion. A paradoxical, and thus falsely localizing, ipsilateral hemiparesis may also occur because the herniation effect of the uncus may exert pressure not only downward but also across the midbrain. On the other side, the edge of the tentorium cerebelli may be pressed against the contralateral cerebral peduncle at the area of a bony prominence. This leads to an indentation of the cerebral peduncle known as Kernohan's notch. Hence, the very lateral corticospinal tracks may be pressed contralateral to the side of uncal herniation, leading actually to an early hemiparesis ipsilateral to the lesion. In uncal herniation, the side of the lesion localizes reliably to the side of the dilated pupil but not necessarily to the side of the hemiparesis!

Ischemia to the nerve can also occur

- The blood supply to the nerve is from the vasa nervorum, a network of small perforating vessels feeding the CN III nerve trunk from the outside inward.
- The innermost fibers of the nerve trunk are the most susceptible to ischemia.
- The fibers to the extraocular muscles are concentrated on the inside of the nerve trunk (remember, pupillary constrictor fibers are distributed around the external perimeter of the nerve trunk).
- In an intrinsic (e.g., vasculitic) lesion of CN III, pupillary fibers are spared whereas the fibers to the extraocular muscles (EOMs) and levator muscle are affected.
- Therefore, limitation of eye movement (especially adduction) and ptosis (eyelid droop) can be seen, with normal pupil size, in intrinsic (noncompressive) CN III lesions. The eye may be abducted due to unopposed action of the lateral rectus muscle (CN VI).
- This would be a common finding in diabetes mellitus due to microangiopathy.
- Ophthalmoplegic migraine is a reversible cause.

Muscle disorders

Muscle disorders, or disorders of the neuromuscular junction such as myasthenia, can sometimes mimic the eye movement abnormalities and ptosis seen in oculomotor palsy.

4. Trochlear Nerve—CN IV

Anatomy

- CN IV crosses dorsally and exits from the dorsal brainstem on the opposite side.
- Innervates the superior oblique muscle that turns and moves the eye down when adducted.
- This nerve really helps walking down steps without tripping!

Pathology

- Most commonly affected cranial nerve in head trauma due to shearing forces.
- Etiologies of lesions
  - Trauma
  - Neoplasm
  - Infection
  - Aneurysm
- Patient may tilt head to compensate for diplopia. There is vertical diplopia in CN IV palsy and, in severe weakness, hypertropia (elevation

of the eye in the vertical axis) can also be present. There may also be extorsion (outward rotation of the upper pole) of the eye that usually is not ascertained by the examiner. Head tilt away from the affected eye corrects for this extorsion.

5. Abducens Nerve—CN VI

Anatomy

- Nucleus located in pons (Figure 2.34)
- Passes along base of brain
- Then passes through the cavernous sinus
- Exits skull through the superior orbital fissure and innervates the lateral rectus muscle

> CN III and CN IV reach the eye through the superior orbital fissure. CN II reaches the eye through the optic canal along with the ophthalmic artery and the sympathetic pupillodilator fibers.

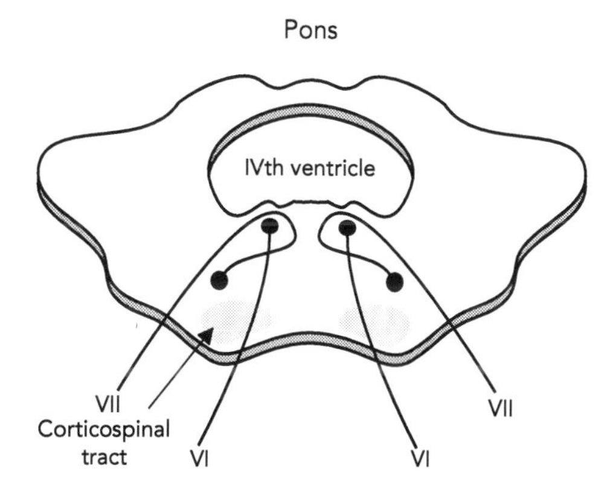

Figure 2.34 The nucleus for CN VI is located in the pons. The nerve passes along the base of the brain and then through the cavernous sinus to exit the skull at the superior orbital fissure. Note that CN VII passes dorsally over the nucleus of CN VI.

Control of Gaze

Conjugate gaze refers to the symmetrical and synchronous movement of the eyes in the same direction. Each eye must move at the same velocity to keep the images on the exact same portion of the retina, preventing double vision.

- Conjugate vertical gaze:
  - CN III controls vertical gaze (Figure 2.35).
  - Right and left CN III are connected via the posterior commissure.

- Tumors pressing on posterior commissure (e.g., pinealoma) may disturb vertical gaze and cause tonic downward deviation of the eyes (Parinaud syndrome).

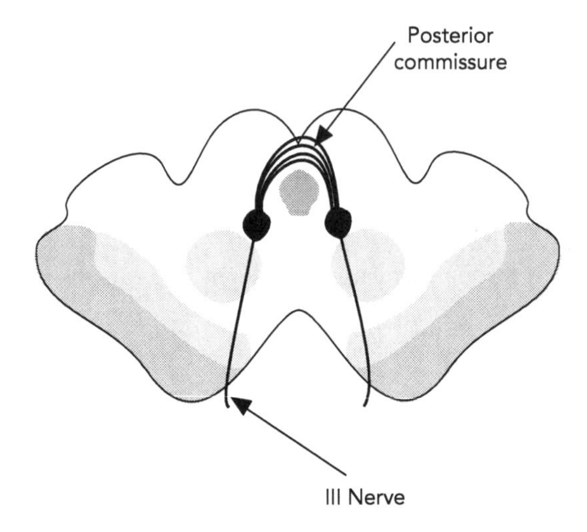

Figure 2.35 A pinealoma or other tumor pressing on the posterior commissure may affect vertical gaze and lead to tonic downward deviation of the eyes.

Conjugate horizontal gaze

- In order to look to the right, the right lateral rectus (CN VI) and the left medial rectus (CN III) muscles are used (Figure 2.36). These are connected via the medial longitudinal fasciculus (MLF), a heavily myelinated, rapidly conducting pathway.
- The abducens nucleus (CN VI) and the essentially contiguous paramedian pontine reticular formation (PPRF) control horizontal movement of both eyes by serving as the horizontal gaze center. Thus, some neurons in the abducens nucleus project to the ipsilateral lateral rectus muscle and others project via the MLF to the contralateral oculomotor nucleus, which in turn activates the contralateral medial rectus muscle. There are two major stimuli for conjugate horizontal gaze:
  - Voluntary influence
  - Vestibular influence

Voluntary influence on gaze

- To look left, the right frontal eye field (Brodmann area 8) is activated (Figure 2.37).
- Impulses travel through corticobulbar tracts—cortical motor fibers descending to the cranial nerves—and cross to the left CN VI nucleus. Thus, the left eye is abducted to the left.

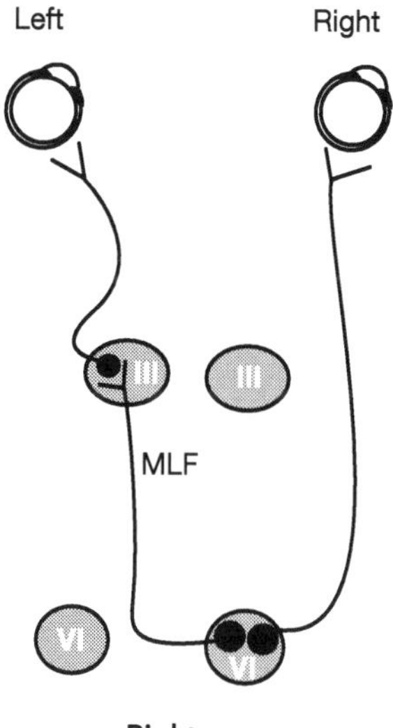

Figure 2.36 The basic brainstem pathway mediating horizontal gaze utilizes the medial longitudinal fasciculus (MLF) to connect the nuclei of cranial nerves III and VI.

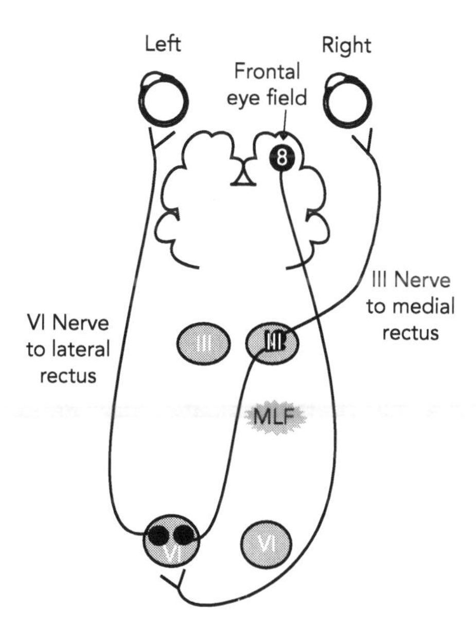

Figure 2.37 Demonstration of how **left** conjugate gaze is achieved. A stimulus from the right frontal lobe (principally the frontal eye field or Brodmann area 8) energizes the contralateral (left) CN VI nucleus serving along with the neighboring PPRF (paramedian pontine reticular formation) as the horizontal gaze center. This causes left eye (OS) abduction as well as contralateral right eye (OD) adduction via the MLF.

- MLF is activated stimulating right medial rectus. Thus, the right eye is adducted, moving it to the left. Hence, conjugate gaze to the left has been achieved!

Vestibular influence on gaze

- Vestibular information enters the MLF from CN VIII to keep the environment stable without ocular blurring despite head movement.
- This is a crossed pathway; the left CN VIII stimulates the right CN VI/ PPRF resulting in right gaze (Figure 2.38).

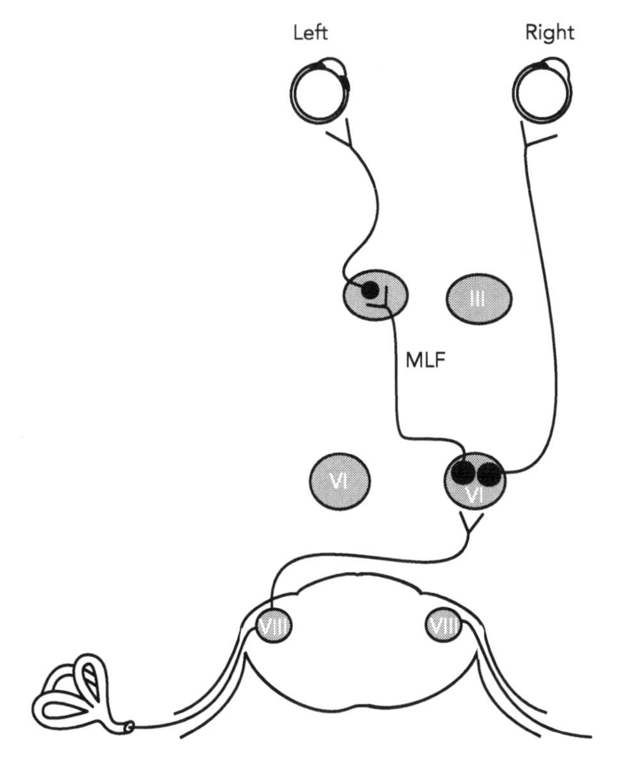

Figure 2.38 Vestibular influence on conjugate gaze involves a crossed pathway; the left CN VIII stimulates the right CN VI/PPRF resulting in right gaze.

Pathology

Cranial nerve VI palsy creates horizontal diplopia that patients describe as better when viewing near objects and worse when viewing far objects.

- Pons:
    - Vascular infarction is associated with:
        - Facial palsy on same side due to CN VII involvement
        - Hemiparesis on opposite side

- May have associated ipsilateral gaze plegia due to involvement of the brainstem gaze center in the region of the CN VI nucleus (see Stroke below).
- Tumor may also cause CN VI palsy in the pons.

■ Nerve:

- Due to its long course, CN VI is susceptible to the effects of increased intracranial pressure. Abducens nerve palsy is therefore an early sign of supratentorial or infratentorial tumors, hydrocephalus, pseudotumor cerebri, or other causes of increased intracranial pressure.
- CN VI is also damaged by processes affecting the subarachnoid space, cavernous sinus, or orbit.
- Many cases cannot be attributed to a particular cause, and may simply be the result of microvascular neuropathy as seen in diabetes mellitus.

■ Stroke (Figure 2.39):

- Stroke may destroy one frontal eye field (right) leaving the other (left) unopposed and resulting in *right* tonic eye deviation and loss of gaze to the left. This is known as a right gaze preference or left gaze palsy.
- Seizures may stimulate one eye field (right) resulting in *left* tonic eye deviation.
- A brainstem stroke in the region of the CN VI nucleus may also result in eye deviation, but this time ipsiversive gaze (i.e., toward the same side) is lost, and hence the eyes look *away* from the brainstem stroke. Note that this contrasts with gaze deviation following a cortical stroke where the eyes look toward the infarcted side.

A right pontine stroke, however, may result in decreased activity of the right horizontal gaze center (PPRF), causing loss of ipsiversive (right) gaze and resultant gaze deviation away from the stroke (i.e., to the left). Thus, the eyes look toward a cortical stroke but away from a brainstem stroke. The PPRF is wrapped around the CN VI nucleus; hence, lesions at the pontine level manifest as gaze palsies rather than an isolated CN VI palsy.

■ Nystagmus:

Dysfunction of the labyrinth results in *nystagmus*, an unstable jerky eye movement, along with nausea and vomiting. The integrity of the labyrinths and this pathway can be tested clinically by the:

- Oculocephalic reflex (doll's eye manuever)
- Oculovestibular reflex (calorics, used when a stimulus stronger than the doll's eye maneuver is needed)

In the case of the doll's eyes, the eyes floating from side to side in the globe in response to movement of the head should be seen like in the expensive dolls in the store—not like in the cheap dolls where the eyes are drawn

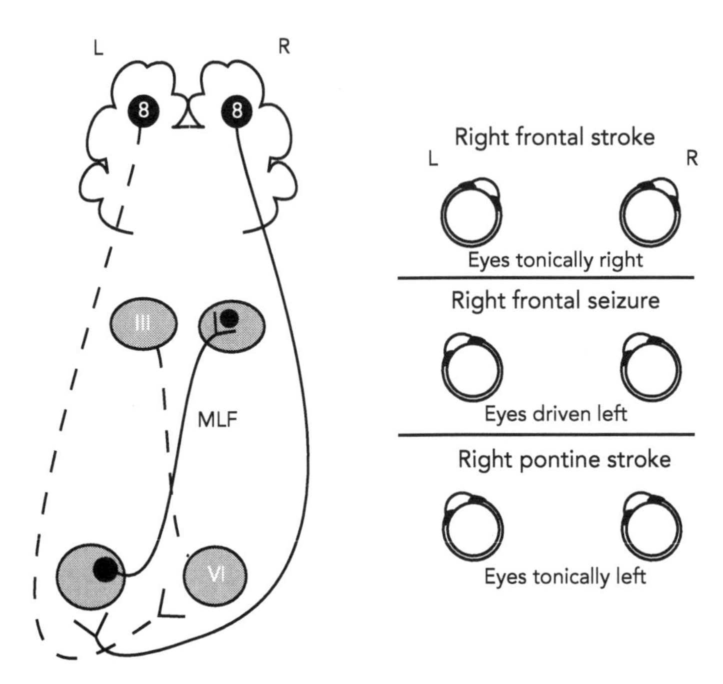

Figure 2.39 There is a dynamic balance of the input from the right and left frontal eye fields. A right frontal stroke leads to loss of baseline stimulation from the right frontal cortical eye field, leaving unopposed action of the intact left frontal eye field. Thus, the eyes deviate to the right (toward the cortical stroke). Conversely, a right frontal seizure may activate the pathway, driving the eyes to the left.

on and are fixed in position. Normally when the head moves to the right the eyes move a proportionate distance to the left so that external focus may be maintained and objects in extracorporeal space do not appear to move.

In the case of calorics, ice cold water will inhibit the neural transmission from the CN VIII nucleus to the contralateral CN VI nucleus and surrounding PPRF. Thus, this influence on conjugate gaze is lost, and the unopposed baseline activity from the other side compensates by pushing the eyes the other way. Hence, it is *normal* for the eyes to drive *toward* the ice. It means the other side of the brainstem is working, all the way from the contralateral CN VIII nucleus at the pontomedullary junction to the corresponding CN VI nucleus/PPRF, and up to the origin of the MLF in the midbrain (Figure 2.40).

Note that ice cold water is used during the coma examination to achieve the strongest stimulus possible to test the integrity of the brainstem. In the evaluation of an awake patient with vertigo, cool water (30°C) or warm water (44°C) can be used. In that case, the eyes still deviate toward the cool water because of the pathways above. But the patient who is awake will show a rapidly corrective nystagmus that goes the *opposite* way from the water. It is basically the brain's way of saying, "Get your eyes back on the road!" Since nystagmus is named for that fast phase, the mnemonic COWS (cold, opposite; warm, same) is true. Keep in mind that this mnemonic is not helpful in a coma where there is no corrective nystagmus and the eyes remain deviated!

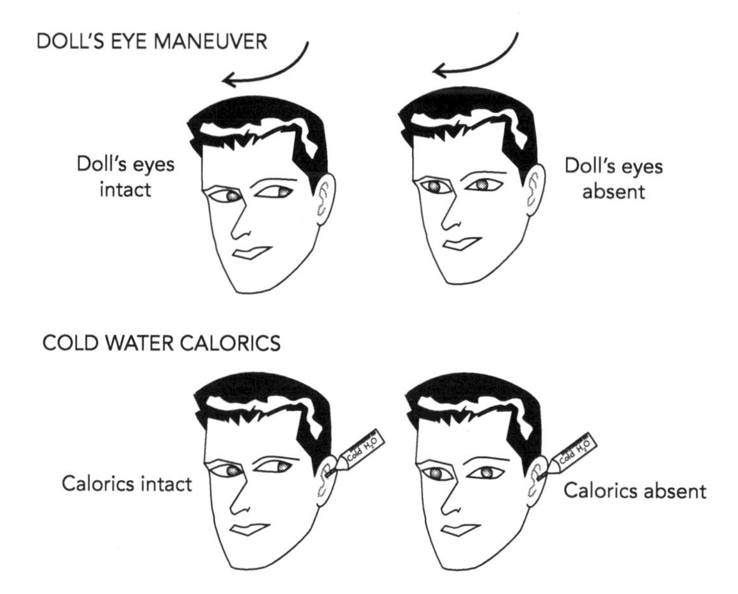

Figure 2.40 In the "doll's" eye maneuver (oculocephalic reflex), the eyes should float in their sockets with head movement. In the cold water calorics maneuver (vestibulo-ocular reflex), the eyes normally should deviate toward the side of the water. Cold water inhibits firing in the pathway leaving the unopposed action of the intact side. If the doll's eye maneuver is intact, then there is no need to do cold water calorics. Cold water is a more vigorous stimulus to the same pathway.

> Clinical Pearl
>
> Here is another trick to distinguish cortical versus brainstem strokes: One would not be able to overcome the gaze plegia in the pontine stroke through the "doll's" eye/oculocephalic maneuver because the horizontal gaze center is lesioned. In contrast, the gaze preference toward a cortical lesion can be overcome with this bedside maneuver.

- Disorders of the MLF:
  - Interruption of the MLF results in dysconjugate gaze—internuclear ophthalmoplegia (INO) (Figure 2.41). That is, there is a lesion between the nuclei resulting in extraocular motor weakness or paralysis.
  - In the classic INO, there is failure of adduction on the side of the lesion when attempting horizontal gaze and corresponding nystagmus of the opposite eye. The latter is known as abduction nystagmus.

- The INO manifests as double vision (diplopia) during horizontal gaze.
- Etiologies:
  - Demyelinating plaque, as in multiple sclerosis
  - Small vessel infarction

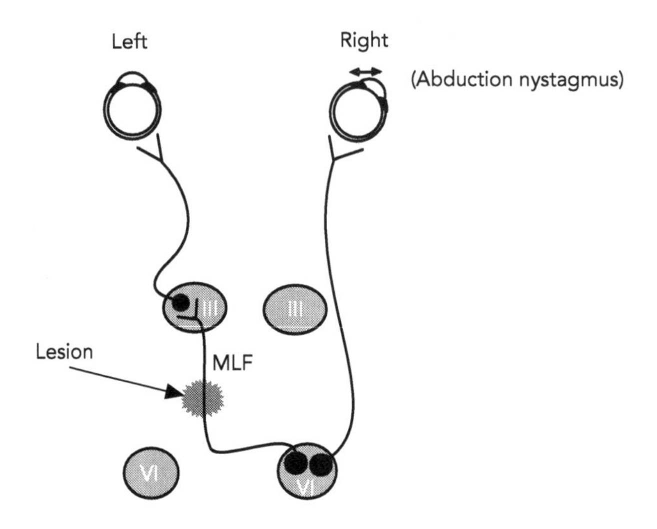

Figure 2.41 Destruction of the MLF results in an INO (internuclear opthalmoplegia). This is manifest by loss of adduction of the eye ipsilateral to the lesion, and nystagmus on abduction of the other eye. Associated symptoms are severe double vision (diplopia), nausea, and dizziness.

6. Trigeminal Nerve—CN V

Anatomy (Figure 2.42)

As its name implies, this nerve has three major branches: the ophthalmic division (V1), maxillary division (V2), and mandibular division (V3). The trigeminal nerve provides sensory innervation to the face. The sensory nucleus of the trigeminal nerve is the largest cranial nerve nucleus. Cranial nerve V also has a small motor nucleus that is responsible for controlling the muscles of mastication (masseter and temporalis muscles) and some other small muscles (tensor tympani, tensor veli palatine, mylohyoid, and anterior belly of digastric).

Pathology

Clinically, most disorders of CN V function produce facial numbness or tingling paresthesias. Demonstrable weakness in the muscles of mastication is unusual.

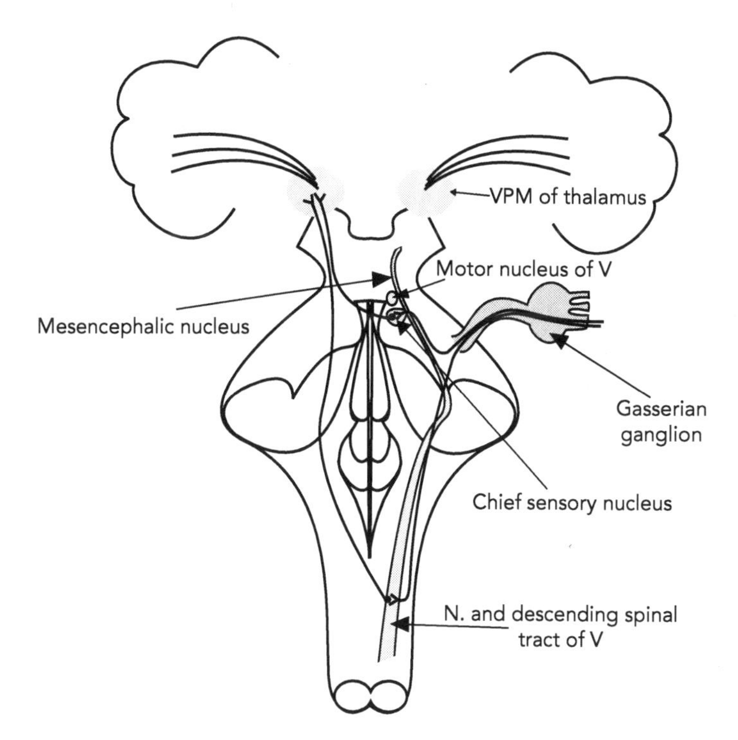

Figure 2.42 Cranial nerve V, the trigeminal nerve, descends from its nucleus in the pons down to the upper cervical spinal cord as the descending tract and nucleus of CN V. Secondary trigeminal fibers from the spinal tract nucleus cross to the other side and ascend up the medial lemniscus, to synapse in the VPM (ventroposteromedial) nucleus of the thalamus.

- Cortex (postcentral gyrus):
  - Numbness and tingling of opposite side of face
  - Etiology: stroke, tumor, hemorrhage, abscess

- Thalamus:
  - More substantial loss of all sensory modalities to opposite side of face as fibers are consolidated at this level
  - Etiology: stroke, tumor, hemorrhage, abscess (same as above)

- Brainstem:
  - Most commonly involves the descending spinal tract of CN V (pain and temperature) due to its peripheral location
  - Decreased sensation to pinprick over the ipsilateral face
  - Often associated sensory loss on contralateral body due to involvement of medial lemniscus; hence, crossed findings (ipsilateral facial and contralateral body)
  - Etiology: brainstem vascular insufficiency or infarction

- Base of the brain:
  - Compression by tumor, especially acoustic neuroma in cerebellopontine angle associated with initial CNs VII and VIII involvement
  - Entrapment in cavernous sinus secondary to cavernous sinus thrombosis (V1 and V2)
  - Gasserian ganglion itself may be involved with herpes zoster (painful herpetic eruption on same side of face)

- Clinical application—trigeminal neuralgia (tic douloureux):
  - Brief lancinating facial pain (fleeting but excruciating)
  - Usually maxillary (V2) or mandibular (V3) division
  - Middle-aged or older
  - Etiology: idiopathic but underlying causes include multiple sclerosis, brainstem infarction, tumor of the cerebellopontine angle (CPA, see below under CN VII), aberrant superior cerebellar artery resting on the nerve
  - Treatment—antiepileptic medications, for example, carbamazepine, oxcarbazepine, and neurosurgical procedures (insertion of cotton pledget between nerve and vessel as well as ablative procedures)

Abducens Nerve—CN VI

Highlights: The abducens nerve innervates the lateral rectus muscle, is frequently affected as a nonlocalizing sign in many causes of increased intracranial pressure, and is covered earlier with cranial nerves III and IV in the section on extraocular muscles.

7. Facial Nerve—CN VII

As its name implies, the facial nerve primarily serves to control the muscles of facial expression; however, it has other functions as well.

Anatomy

The main nerve trunk carries the motor fibers controlling facial expression, whereas a smaller branch called the nervus intermedius carries fibers for the parasympathetic (tears and salivation), special sensory (taste), and general somatosensory (sensation to the external auditory canal and skin behind the ear) functions (see Figure 2.43). In the brainstem, the roots coming off the CN VII nucleus ascend to the level of the CN VI nucleus, and sweep over the abducens nuclei as the genu of the facial nerve. The nerve then exits the ventrolateral pons.

Multiple components and functions

- Branchial motor: muscles of facial expression (and stapedius, stylohyoid, posterior belly of digastric, buccinators, platysma, occipitalis)

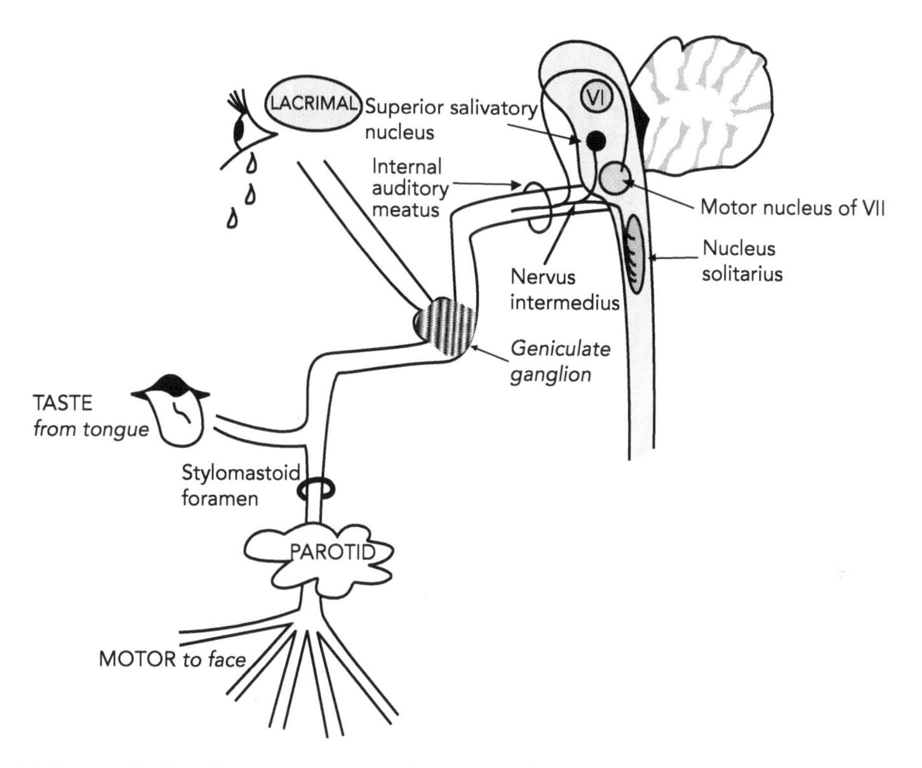

Figure 2.43 The nervus intermedius carries fibers for parasympathetic, special sensory, and general somatosensory functions.

- Visceral motor: lacrimal, submandibular, sublingual glands, mucous membrane of nose and palate (hard and soft)
- General somatosensory: external auditory canal, skin just behind the ear
- Special sensory: taste from anterior two-thirds of tongue and hard and soft palate

Central versus peripheral patterns of facial weakness

The facial nerve fibers allow one to wrinkle the brow (frontalis muscle), close the eye and even bury the lids together (orbicularis oculi), and close the mouth (orbicularis oris). Note that frontalis function (eyebrow wrinkling) is often referred to the upper face (or upper one-third, sometimes loosely called the upper half), and eyelid and mouth closure belong to the lower face.

The traditional teaching that supranuclear innervation to the face is bilateral to the frontalis fibers (upper one-third) and strictly contralateral to the lower two-thirds of the face appears to be more dogmatic than truth. Anatomical studies instead demonstrate a gradient where there is less cortical innervation to the forehead, that is, the frontalis fibers receive less attention from higher centers, not more. In any case, the key clinicoanatomic correlation is that supranuclear lesions, that is, lesions above the facial nerve nucleus, cause weakness of the contralateral lower face (sparing the upper one-third frontalis fibers, or eyebrow wrinkling). In contrast, lesions of the facial nerve nucleus in the pons or the actual cranial nerve cause a more severe and full deficit affecting the entire (upper and lower) ipsilateral facial muslces.

Pathology

- Supranuclear lesions:

  A supranuclear lesion causing facial weakness, located above the level of the CN VII nucleus in the pons, causes a more subtle and less complete deficit. That is, the contralateral facial weakness is limited to the lower two thirds of the face, and is less severe than the weakness seen in a lesion affecting the nucleus or exiting cranial nerve.

  Central facial weakness can be on the basis of either a volitional or mimetic deficit. Volitional paresis (i.e., inability to intentionally move the face or respond to a command to smile) indicates cortical involvement of the contralateral precentral gyrus, internal capsule, cerebral peduncle, or upper pons. Mimetic or emotional paresis (i.e., inability to show a reflexive emotional facial response, or smile fully at a funny joke) indicates a lesion typically involving the thalamus or insula.

- Nuclear and peripheral cranial nerve VII lesions:

  These involve the complete ipsilateral hemiface (upper and lower muscles). The severity of the weakness is typically more dense weakness, at least early in the course. There is no dissociation here between volitional and reflexive facial movements.

  - Brainstem lesion

    Figure 2.44 shows a pontine lesion that leads to complete right facial paralysis. In this case, the actual cranial nerve VII nucleus is involved, so it is really a nuclear facial palsy and has the same features as the peripheral cranial neuropathy, with the complete face involved (upper and lower facial muscles). In addition, there are other deficits due to the involvement of neighboring structures:

    - Right complete facial weakness
    - Loss of gaze to the right (due to involvement of the right PPRF)
    - Left hemiparesis (due to involvement of the descending corticospinal tract in the ventral pons, which will eventually cross in the decussation of the pyramids in the ventral medulla caudally)

  - Cerebellopontine angle (CPA): a dangerous corner (as in 3rd base)

    - Compression of CN VII by tumor (Figure 2.45)
      - Especially vestibular schwannoma (aka acoustic neuroma)
      - Associated tinnitus and hearing loss
      - Peripheral facial palsy on same side

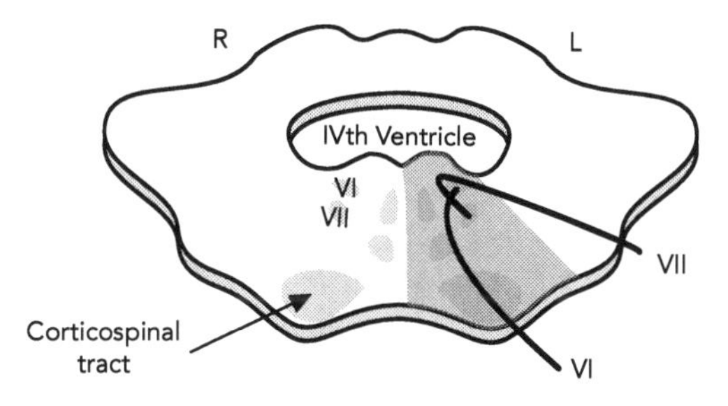

Figure 2.44 Note how a pontine lesion will affect the complete face (both upper and lower facial muscles) and neighboring structures, such as CN VI and the descending corticospinal tract in the ventral pons. This may be seen due to infarction of a small paramedian basilar artery perforating branch that supplies this discrete territory or with invasive brainstem tumor

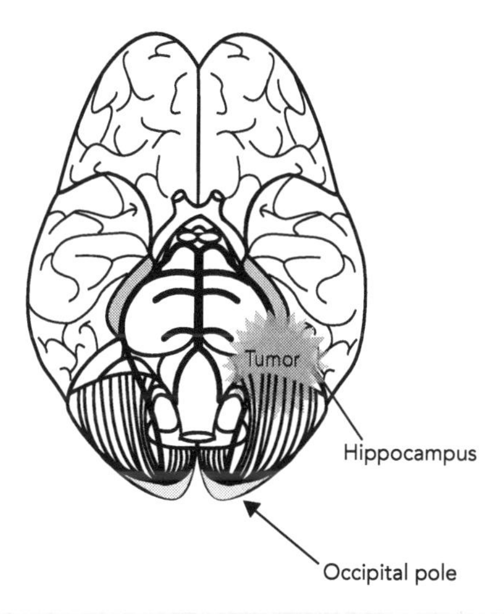

Figure 2.45 Compression of CN VII and VIII by a tumor at the cerebellopontine angle (CPA) can cause CPA syndrome, which may manifest as tinnitus, hearing loss, ataxia, vertigo, and ipsilateral peripheral facial nerve palsy.

- Basilar meningitis may entrap the nerve and cause a CPA syndrome
  - Fungal, syphilitic, or tuberculous meningitis
  - Sarcoidosis

- Internal auditory canal
  - Compression by tumor, especially vestibular schwannoma
  - Associated loss of lacrimation, taste, and salivation may occur, as well as hyperacusis (due to involvement of the nerve to the stapedius muscle, which ordinarily tightens the ossicles of the ear and protects from loud noises)

- Facial canal to stylomastoid foramen
  - Viral, postviral, or idiopathic processes affect the nerve here secondary to swelling and nerve compression, leading to peripheral facial palsy (Bell's palsy) (Figure 2.46)
  - Lacrimation, salivation, and taste may be involved
  - More than 80% of cases of Bell's palsy have a full spontaneous recovery

Bell's palsy, is named for Sir Charies Bell: Scottish surgeon, anatomist, philosophical theologian, 1774–1842.

Note: The most common cause of bilateral CN VII palsy is Lyme disease.

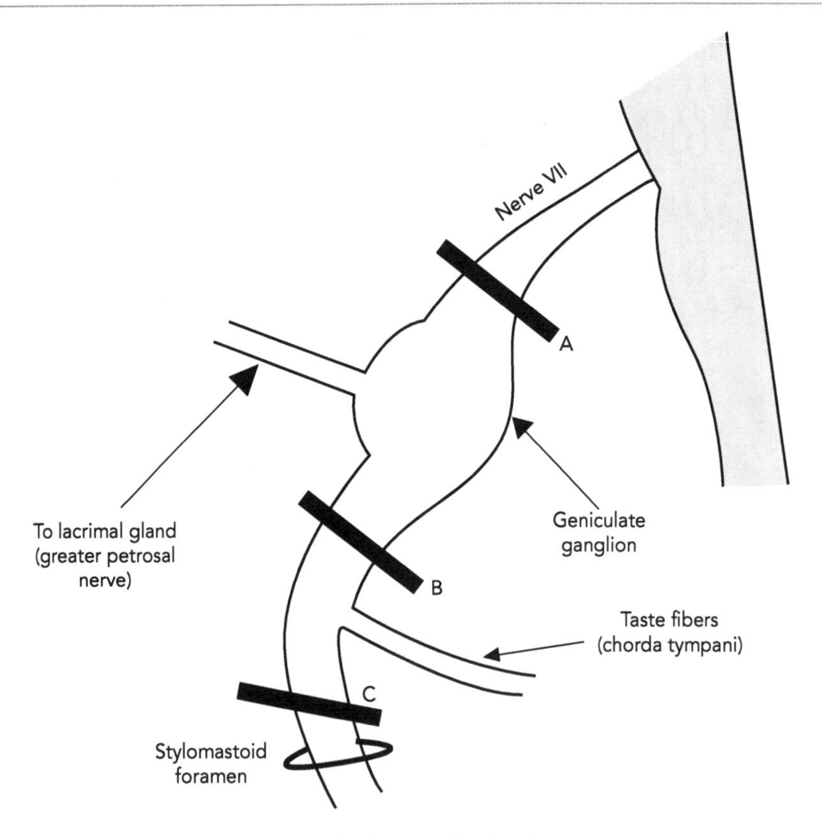

Figure 2.46 There are several potential sites of lesions causing Bell's palsy, generating progressively more symptoms as the lesion moves proximally.

Anatomical detail of the intracranial branches of CN VII: The greater petrosal nerve carries parasympathetic fibers to the lacrimal gland. The nerve to the stapedius (not shown in Figure 2.46) supplies motor innervation to the stapedius muscle. The chorda tympani carry taste fibers from the anterior two thirds of the tongue and innervation to the sublingual and submandibular salivary glands.

Clinical application: special disorders associated with peripheral facial palsy

- Herpes zoster of the geniculate ganglion:
  - Herpetic vesicular eruption in the external auditory canal
  - Accompanying ipsilateral facial palsy
- Parotid gland lesions:
  - Inflammatory (parotitis)
  - Neoplasms
  - Postsurgical

8. Acoustic/Vestibular Nerve—CN VIII

Anatomy

The nucleus for CN VIII is located at the pontomedullary junction, and is actually composed of several nuclei. The cranial nerve itself enters the internal auditory meatus in the temporal bone and enters the brainstem through the cerebellopontine angle (CPA). This is a sensory nerve that carries auditory information from the cochlea and balance information from the vestibular apparatus.

Once the CN VIII fibers from the cochlea and vestibular apparatus synapse in the vestibulocochlear nuclei of the brainstem, the majority cross to the superior olivary complex and ascend through the lateral lemniscus. These fibers synapse in the inferior colliculus of the dorsal tectum of the midbrain. They proceed to the medial geniculate body of the thalamus and, after synapsing, emerge as the thalamocortical projections to eventually reach Heschl's gyri (Brodmann area 41, 42). Some fibers, however, do not cross in the brainstem, and ascend through the ipsilateral lateral lemniscus to reach the ipsilateral Heschl's gyrus. Hence, hearing is represented bilaterally in the brain.

Pathology

- Lesions of the cochlear/vestibular apparatus:
  - Congenital lesions (deafness)
  - Acquired lesions
    - Tinnitus (ringing in ear)
    - Hearing loss

    - Vertigo (unsteadiness)
    - Nausea and vomiting
    - Etiologies: viral labyrinthitis, Ménière's disease (endolymphatic hydrops)

- CPA and internal auditory canal:
  - Associated deficits of CNs V, VI, VII, IX, X, and XI may occur.
  - Deafness is a common sequela of purulent meningitis in children.
  - Neurofibromatosis type 2 is characterized by bilateral acoustic/vestibular schwannomas and a chromosome 22 deletion.

- Brainstem:
  - Disruption of cochlear and vestibular nuclei cause less clear-cut symptoms than the more peripheral lesions described earlier.
  - Associated neighborhood signs occur depending on the extent of the brainstem lesion.

- Cortical lesions:
  - Rarely associated with deafness, unless there is extensive bilateral involvement. This is known as cortical deafness.
  - Temporal lobe seizures
    - Vertiginous sensation as aura (warning phase preceding a seizure)
    - Auditory hallucination as aura
  - Auditory agnosias may occur secondary to a unilateral lesion of the dominant posterior temporal cortex, or bilateral temporal lesions affecting Heschl's gyri. One example is pure word deafness, which is the inability to understand spoken language despite normal auditory acuity, reading, writing, naming, and comprehension of non-language sounds.

9. Glossopharyngeal Nerve—CN IX

This nerve deals with the tongue (glossus) and the pharynx.

Anatomy

- CN IX is primarily a sensory nerve, providing sensory information from the posterior third of the tongue, external ear, and tympanic membrane, and taste from the posterior third of the tongue. (Note that the trigeminal nerve, CN V3, contributes sensation from the anterior two-thirds of the tongue, and the facial nerve, CN VII, contributes taste information from the anterior two-thirds of the tongue.)
- CN IX contributes to salivation and swallowing, and also receives input from the baroreceptors of the carotid sinus (monitoring blood

pressure) and chemoreceptors of the carotid body (monitoring CO_2 and O_2 concentrations).

- Supranuclear innervation to CN IX is bilateral.

Pathology

- It is unusual to find an isolated lesion of CN IX, due to its close anatomical association with CNs X and XI. A pure glossopharyngeal syndrome consists of loss of the gag reflex (afferent arc mediated by CN IX; efferent arc mediated by CNs IX and X), mild dysphagia, mild palatal droop, and sensory loss involving general sensation of the otorhinolaryngeal area.
- Lesions in the CPA or the jugular foramen may affect CN IX.
- A hypersensitive carotid sinus reflex may cause hypotension, bradycardia, and syncope.

Clinical application: glossopharyngeal neuralgia is a unilateral sharp, stabbing, sudden pain in the throat or ear that lasts seconds to minutes in duration. It is often triggered by chewing, coughing, talking, yawning, swallowing, or tongue protrusion. Sometimes it is more persistent with a dull, aching quality. There may be associated salivation, hoarseness, or syncope. Although usually considered idiopathic (i.e., of unknown cause), lesions along the peripheral glossopharyngeal nerve (e.g., tumor, infection, trauma) or, rarely, a demyelinative plaque in the medulla from multiple sclerosis, should be ruled out. Its analogue is trigeminal neuralgia (see CN V earlier), except that multiple sclerosis is common in trigeminal neuralgia and not in glossopharyngeal neuralgia.

Sidebar Related to the Lower Cranial Nerves

Corticobulbar lesions, distributed bilaterally to the cranial nerve nuclei (in particular CNs VII, IX, and X nuclei and the nucleus ambiguous), may manifest as pseudobulbar palsy. Here, patients show great exaggerated facial movements with pathological laughter and crying, also known as emotional incontinence. This may also result in a spastic tongue and an explosive spastic dysarthria.

10. Vagus Nerve—CN X

This nerve mediates phonation, swallowing (with CNs IX, XI, and XII), taste, cutaneous ear sensation, and elevation of the palate. It also travels or wanders (*vagus* is Latin for wanders) farther to innervate the viscera of the neck, thorax, and abdomen.

Anatomy

- Exits the brainstem from the postolivary sulcus.
- Exits the skull through the jugular foramen with CNs IX and XI.
- The special visceral efferent (SVE), or branchial motor component, originates in the nucleus ambiguous and innervates most of the striated muscles of pharynx and larynx (except the stylopharyngeus and tensor veli palatini).
- The general visceral efferent (GVE), or visceral motor component, originates in the dorsal motor nucleus of the vagus and provides parasympathetic innervation of the viscera of the neck, the heart, and the abdominal cavities down to the left colic flexure.
- The general visceral afferent (GVA) component of the vagus receives sensations from the mucosae of the pharynx, larynx, esophagus, trachea, and thoracic and abdominal viscera, with cell bodies in the inferior vagal ganglion, and transmits this information to the brain via the nucleus of the solitary tract.
- The general somatic afferent (GSA) component has cell bodies in the superior vagal ganglion and carries primary touch, pressure, pain, and temperature sensations from the external acoustic meatus, external tympanic membrane, and pharynx to the brain via the spinal trigeminal tract and nucleus.
- The special visceral afferent (SVA) component has cell bodies in the inferior vagal ganglion (nodose) and carries taste sensation from the epiglottic region to the brain via the nucleus of the solitary tract.

Pathology

- Ipsilateral paralysis, leading to dysphonia, dyspnea, dysarthria and dysphagia, or complete laryngeal paralysis (asphyxia).
- Loss of the gag reflex.
- Anesthesia of the pharynx and larynx, with unilateral loss of cough reflex.
- Cardiac rhythm affections: bradycardia if irritative lesion, tachycardia if destructive lesion.
- Abdominal symptoms, such as impaired gastric emptying (gastroparesis).
- There are two classical vagal reflexes to check CN X's bradycardic response: oculocardiac reflex (pressing the eyes) and the carotid sinus reflex (pressing the carotid sinus).

11. Spinal Accessory Nerve—CN XI

This is a motor nerve that innervates the larynx, head, and shoulders. It has two divisions: cranial and spinal.

Anatomy

- Cranial or accessory portion:
  - Extends from the nucleus ambiguous of the medulla and travels through the postolivary sulcus, joins CN X, and shares the jugular foramen with CNs IX and X.
  - Innervates the intrinsic muscles (except cricothyroid muscle) of the larynx via the recurrent or inferior laryngeal nerve.
- Spinal portion:
  - Extends from the ventral horns of C1 to C6 and ascends through the foramen magnum, and then through the jugular foramen.
  - Innervates the sternocleidomastoid (SCM) muscle (C2) and trapezius (C3–C4).

Pathology

- Paralysis of the larynx if the cranial root is affected.
- Paralysis of the SCM or the trapezius if cervical roots are affected.

12. Hypoglossal Nerve—CN XII

Last, but not least, this cranial nerve mediates tongue movement.

Anatomy

- Extends from the hypoglossal nucleus of the medulla near the midline and traverses the hypoglossal canal to exit the skull.
- Innervates the ipsilateral extrinsic and intrinsic muscles of the tongue.
- Muscles of right side of tongue push the tongue to the left. Need balance of bilateral innervation for the tongue to protrude in the midline.

Pathology

- Hemiparalysis of the tongue if nerve transection occurs.
- Deviation of the protruded tongue to the weak side.

C. THE BASAL GANGLIA: THE TEMPO OF MOVEMENT

The concept of a separate pyramidal (corticospinal) and an extrapyramidal motor system is technically incorrect, since all extrapyramidal influence on motor activity works via its modulation of corticospinal function. It is a functionally useful distinction but it is important to remember that there is no direct motor outflow from the basal ganglia or the cerebellum. These structures influence motor outflow via thalamocortical radiations affecting the net corticospinal outflow.

1. Extrapyramidal System

May be divided into two parts

- Basal ganglia
- Cerebellum

2. Basal Ganglia

Constituents

The basal ganglia, literally nests of neurons sitting at the base of the brain, are composed of the corpus striatum (caudate, putamen), globus pallidus (internal and external portions), and substantia nigra (Figure 2.47). Some would include the subthalamic nucleus, sometimes referred to as the Body of Luys or luysian, which would define the basal ganglia then as "striatopallidonigroluysian." The basal ganglia are key in the modulation of balance and execution of movements, especially previously learned motor movements.

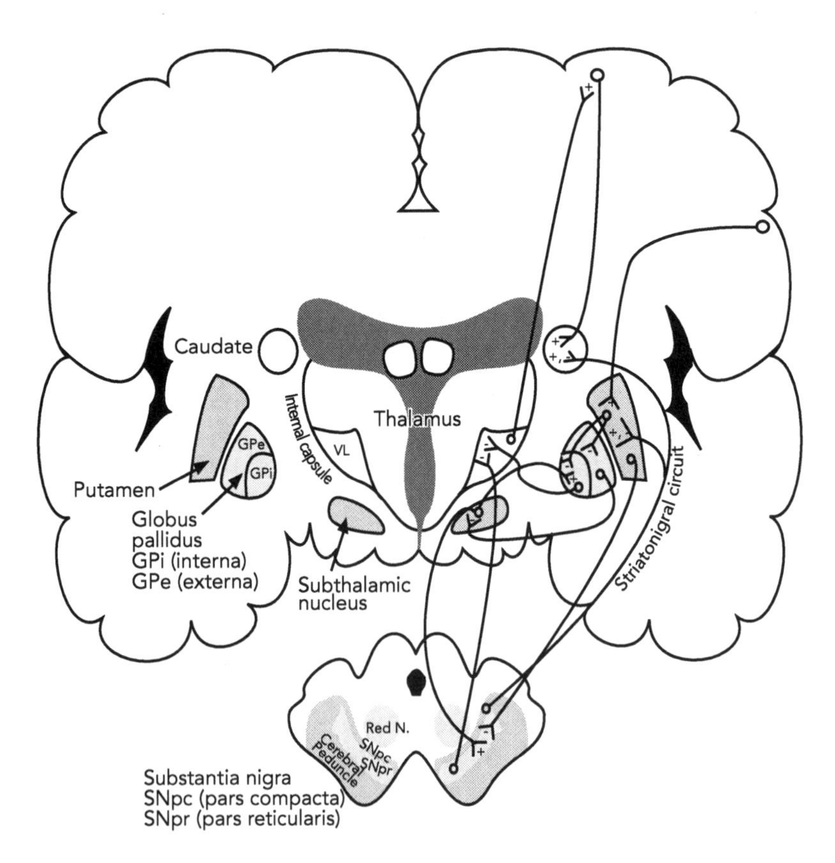

Figure 2.47 Basal ganglia.

Pathway

- The globus pallidus functions as a way station that then funnels information to the ventrolateral (VL) nucleus of the thalamus.
- Information from the VL nucleus of the thalamus is then distributed to diffuse cortical regions.
- There is an additional reciprocal circuit between the striatum (caudate-putamen) and the substantia nigra.
- The VL nucleus of the thalamus (which also receives cerebellar information) is the final common pathway for extrapyramidal information. Information then travels to the cerebral cortex via diffuse thalamocortical radiations.
- Neurotransmitters play a key role in disease processes affecting the basal ganglia, particularly Parkinson disease and Huntington disease.
  - Acetylcholine, GABA (gamma-aminobutyric acid), and dopamine are the primary basal ganglia neurotransmitters, in addition to glutamate and peptides (enkephalin, substance P, and endorphin).

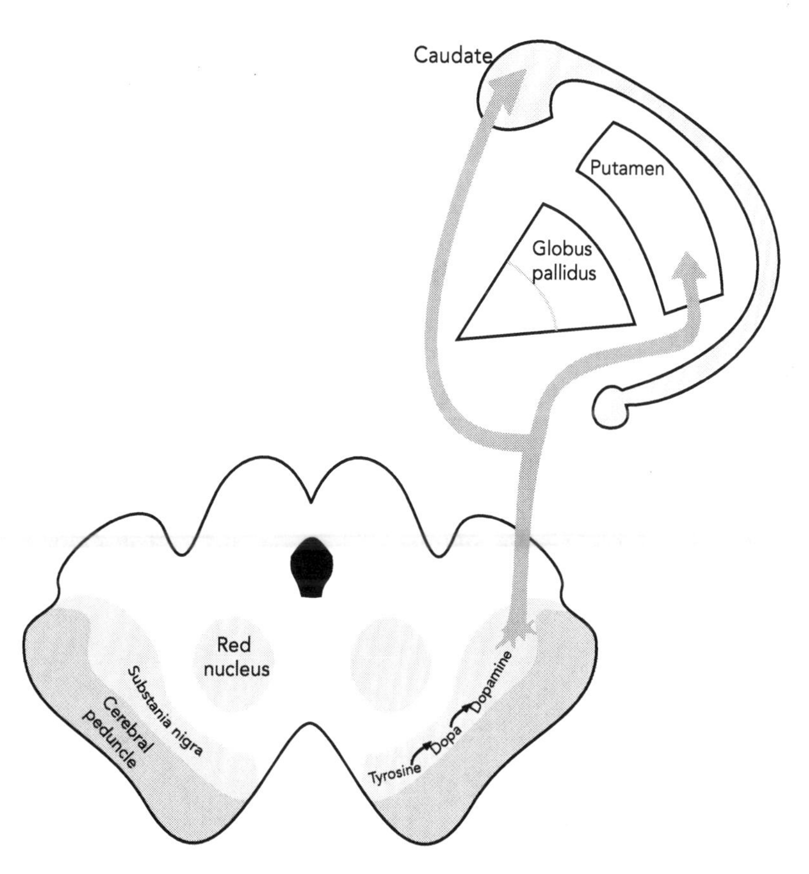

Figure 2.48 Pathway of dopamine synthesis in substantia nigra of the midbrain, with projections to the corpus striatum (caudate and putamen).

- The influences of acetylcholine (excitatory) and dopamine (inhibitory) are balanced to yield normal function.
- Dopamine is manufactured in pigmented nerve cell bodies in the substantia nigra and projected via axons to the corpus striatum (i.e., caudate and putamen) (Figure 2.48). Nerve cell loss in the substantia nigra leads to depletion of dopamine in the striatum, leading to the motor manifestations of Parkinsonism.

The anatomy of the basal ganglia pathways is often mechanistically described as two co-dependent pathways—the *direct* and *indirect* pathways. Overall, the direct pathway results ultimately in increased thalamocortical activity and activation of movement; the indirect pathway results in decreased thalamocortical activity and inhibition of movement. As shown in Figure 2.49, the direct pathway shows the corpus striatum (i.e., caudate and putamen) inhibiting the globus pallidus interna. This results in disinhibition and, hence, activation of the thalamus and then cerebral cortex. Instead, the indirect pathway leads to inhibition of the intermediate globus pallidus externa. This brings about disinhibition of the subthalamic nucleus that then generates further activation of the globus pallidus interna. However, that causes inhibition of the thalamus, and hence decreased thalamocortical and cortical activity.

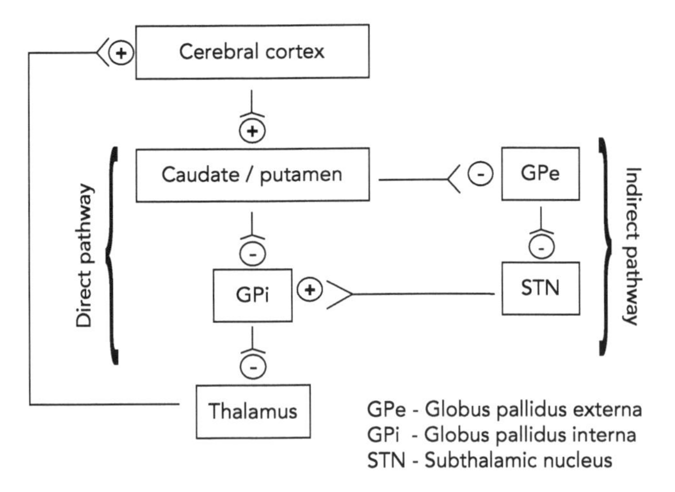

Figure 2.49 Schematic of the direct and indirect pathways of the basal ganglia influencing movement.

Movement disorders

Movement disorders can be viewed in various ways. One way is how the movements themselves appear (i.e., the description of semiology of the movements). Another way is based on the amount and speed of movement (i.e., paucity or excess of movement). Both these paradigms are depicted here.

- Descriptive approach to movement disorders (semiology):
  - Myoclonus: rapid muscle movement, jerklike
  - Tic: abrupt, repetitive, stereotypical, patterned, involuntary, purposeless movements or sounds (i.e., phonations)
  - Stereotypies: stereotypical movements, usually complex and associated with excitement or stress
  - Chorea: dancelike movement, proximal or distal
  - Athetosis: undulating movement, proximal, often coexists with chorea (i.e., choreoathetosis)
  - Ballismus: wind-up or flail movement of the arm, as if pitching a ball
- Functional approach to movement disorders:
  - Hypokinetic: Parkinsonism
  - Hyperkinetic: Huntington chorea, Sydenham chorea, Tourette syndrome

Parkinsonian syndromes

- Clinical features of Parkinsonism:
  - Bradykinesia—poverty and slowness of movement, masklike facies
  - Tremor—4-hertz pill-rolling tremor
  - Rigidity—particularly cogwheel rigidity
  - Postural instability
- Etiologies of Parkinsonism:
  - Parkinson disease (idiopathic, sometimes genetic)
  - Other dementias: corticobasal degeneration, progressive supranuclear palsy (PSP), multisystem atrophy (MSA), Lewy body dementia
  - Postencephalitic (encephalitis lethargica in the early 1900s)
  - Drug induced (e.g., reserpine, haloperidol, phenothiazines, MPTP [drug of abuse])
  - Multiple small infarctions in the region of substantia nigra or striatonigral tracts
- Treatment of Parkinsonism:
  - L-dopa (dopamine cannot cross the blood–brain barrier)
  - Postsynaptic dopamine receptor agonists
  - Anticholinergics

Clinicoanatomical correlations

- Subthalamic nucleus—contralateral hemiballismus
- Anteroventral caudate—contralateral choreoathetosis
- Globus pallidus—contralateral hemi-Parkinsonism, hemidystonia
- Substantia nigra—Parkinsonism
- Pallidal-putamen—falling to the contralateral side (falling log)

D. THE CEREBELLUM: SETTING THE RHYTHM

Function

- Regulation and control of muscle tone
- Coordination of movement
- Control of posture and gait

> As with the basal ganglia, the influence of the cerebellum on motor function is through modulation of descending corticospinal output.

Three Major Anatomical Subdivisions (Figure 2.50)

- Flocculonodular lobe:
  - Teleologically oldest
  - Input from vestibular nuclei
  - Concerned with equilibrium
  - Lesions disturb equilibrium and produce nystagmus

- Anterior lobe (particularly anterior vermis):
  - Input from spinocerebellar tracts
  - Influences posture and tone
  - Lesions produce ataxia of limbs

- Posterior lobe (neocerebellum, cerebellar hemispheres):
  - Input from cortex via corticobulbar fibers—pontine nuclei–basis pontis
  - Concerned with coordination of skilled movements
  - Lesions result in ataxia of trunk, limbs, and hypotonia

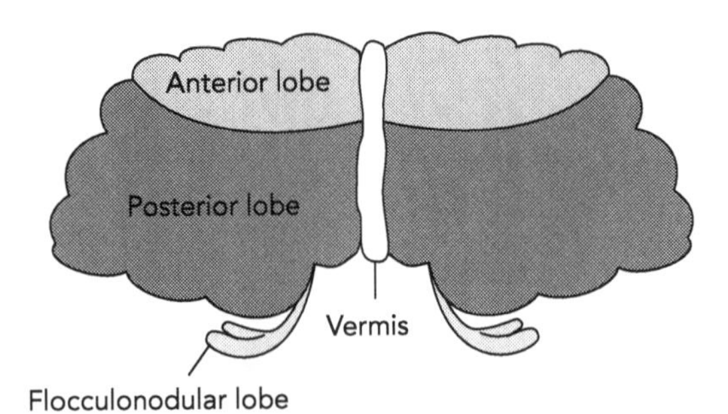

Figure 2.50 The three lobes of the cerebellum. Midline vermis is shown as well.

Three major functional regions (from medial to lateral, based on their input and output connections)

- Vermis and flocculonodular lobe—control of proximal and trunk muscles and vestibulo-ocular control via the:
  - Anterior corticospinal tract, reticulospinal tract, vestibulospinal tract, and tectospinal tract for proximal and trunk muscles
  - Medial longitudinal fasciculus for vestibulo-ocular reflexes
- Intermediate part—control of more distal appendicular muscles via the lateral corticospinal tract and rubrospinal tracts
- Lateral part—motor planning for the extremities via the lateral corticospinal tract

Outputs

- All cerebellar output is relayed by the deep cerebellar nuclei and vestibular nuclei.
- Cerebellar output is all inhibitory.

Pathology

- Ataxia is the cardinal symptom of cerebellar disease, defined as loss of coordination or the smoothness of volitional motor activity.
- Ataxia can affect the limbs (gait disorder or finger-to-nose dysmetria), eyes (jerky eye movements with loss of smooth pursuit), or voice (scanning speech, with long drawn out sounds of varying length).
- Cerebellar lesions are localized based on their own rules:
  - Ataxia is ipsilateral to the side of the cerebellar lesion.
  - Midline lesions of the cerebellar vermis or flocculonodular lobe mainly cause unsteady gait (truncal ataxia) and eye movements, and are often accompanied by intense vertigo, nausea, and vomiting.
  - Lesions lateral to the cerebellar vermis mainly cause ataxia of limbs (appendicular ataxia).
- Examples of pathology affecting the cerebellum:
  - Toxins, especially alcohol (ethanol)
    - Preferentially affects the anterior vermis
    - Related to effects of both alcohol and thiamine (vitamin B_1 deficiency)
    - Predominantly truncal ataxia
  - Infectious
    - Postinfectious (autoimmune)
    - Cerebellar abscess (rare)
  - Neoplastic
    - Primary posterior fossa tumors are common in children (medulloblastoma and cystic astrocytoma).

- Metastases from lung or breast primary tumors.
- Be aware of risk of cerebellar tonsillar herniation, brainstem compression, coma, respiratory arrest, and death from cerebellar structural lesions.

- Vascular disease
  - Hypertensive hemorrhages
    - Be aware of imminent herniation of the cerebellar tonsils due to the proximity of the cerebellum to the foramen magnum.
    - May require emergency evaluation
  - Infarction in anterior inferior cerebellar artery (AICA) or superior cerebellar artery results in hemispheric cerebellar infarct and:
    - Ataxia of ipsilateral limbs
    - Nystagmus
    - Nausea and vomiting occasionally

- Demyelinative disease
  - Multiple sclerosis
  - Acute disseminated encephalomyelitis (ADEM)—postinfectious

- Degenerative disease
  - Olivopontocerebellar atrophy
  - Friedreich ataxia affects the spinocerebellar tracts, lateral corticospinal tracts, and posterior columns (discussed later in the spinal cord section)

> Friedreich ataxia is named for Nikolaus Friedreich: German pathologist and neurologist, 1825–1882.

E. THE SPINAL CORD: THE CNS STOPS HERE

The spinal cord has the cervical (8), thoracic (12), lumbar (5), and sacral (5) segments (Figure 2.51). Although there are eight cervical nerves, there are only seven cervical vertebral bodies. Cervical nerves 1 through 7 exit above their named vertebral bodies, and cervical nerve 8 exits between C7 and T1. All of the remaining segments have the same number of vertebral bodies and nerves, and the nerves exit below their named vertbral bodies. The spinal cord gray matter has the dorsal and ventral horns, and the anterior horn cells in the ventral gray horn represent the prototypical lower motor neuron (LMN). Motor deficits on the neurological examination are often interpreted as representing upper motor neuron (UMN) lesions versus LMN lesions, resulting in UMN and LMN syndromes. The cardinal features of each are summarized in the informal table that follows.

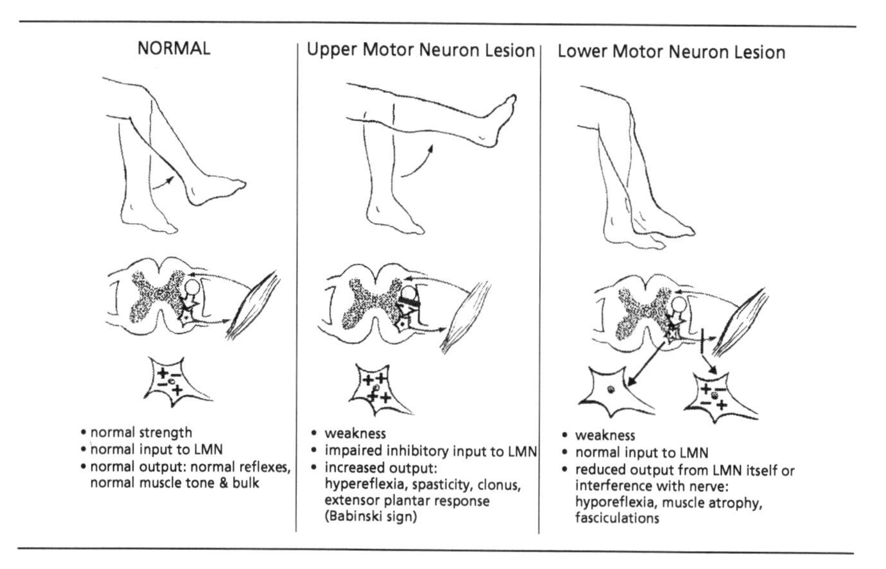

A lesion of the brain or long tracts of the spinal cord, prior to the synapse on the anterior horn cell, is a UMN lesion leading to a UMN syndrome. A lesion of the motor unit (i.e., LMN in the spinal cord, nerve root, peripheral nerve, neuromuscular junction, or muscle within the peripheral nervous system[PNS]) is a LMN lesion and leads to a LMN syndrome. The long white matter tracts of the spinal cord include both descending motor tracts and ascending sensory tracts. The distribution of a spinal cord lesion determines what tracts, and hence clinical deficits, are involved.

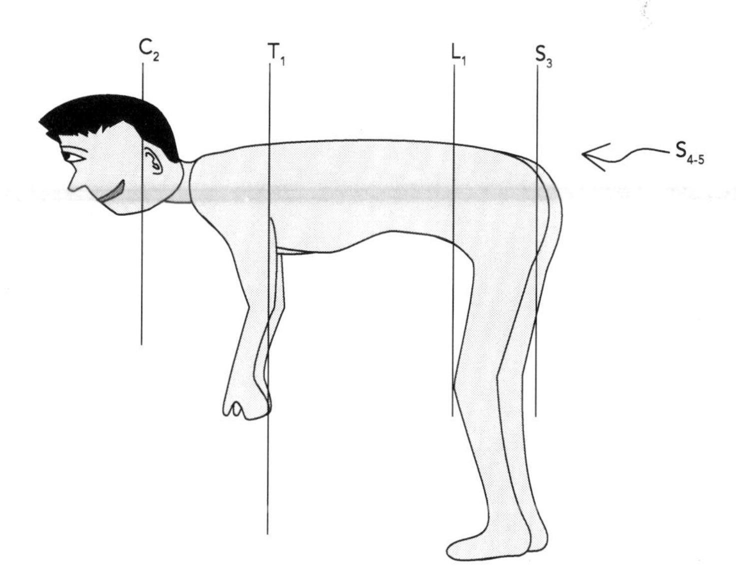

Figure 2.51 Organization of the spinal cord segments.

A side note on terminology: Some investigators prefer the term *motor neuron* for LMN and *premotor neuron* for UMN. The motor neuron is the primary motor neuron of the spinal cord and brainstem that directly innervates muscle, leading to movement. The premotor neurons send descending commands to the motor neurons.

These spinal cord syndromes are depicted in Figure 2.52:

- Tabetic syndrome (dorsal horn)
- Complete transection
- Hemisection/Brown-Sequard syndrome
- Syringomyelia (central cavity)
- Anterior spinal artery syndrome
- Combined degeneration (posterior columns + lateral corticospinal tracts)

1. Complete Transection

- Clinical features (see Figure 2.53):
  - Total loss of sensation *below* the level of the lesion
  - Loss of motor control *below* the level of the lesion
    - Flaccid paralysis with atrophy *at* the lesion level due to destruction of anterior horn cells (LMN effect)
    - Spasticity *below* the level of the lesion due to interference with descending corticospinal tracts (UMN effect)
  - Decrease in voluntary bowel and bladder control
  - Decrease in respiration if lesion is *above* C5 (phrenic nerve to diaphragm is from levels C3–C5)

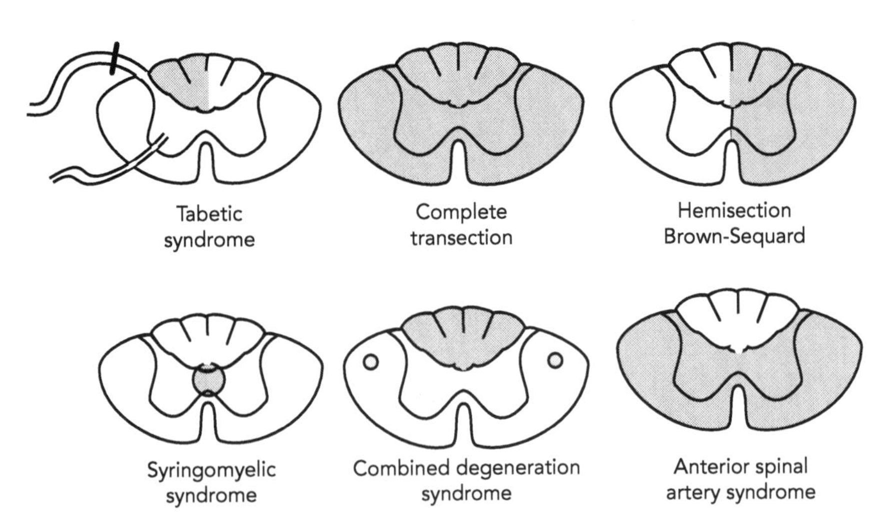

Figure 2.52 Spinal cord syndromes.

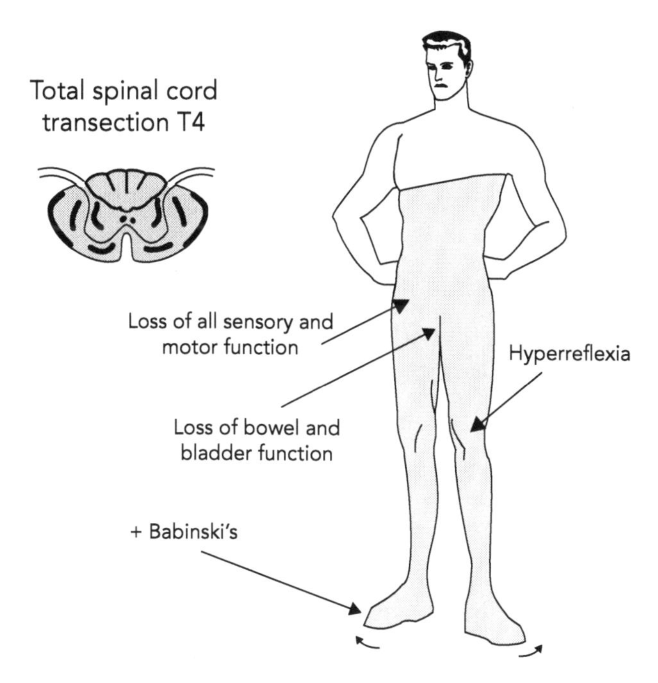

Figure 2.53 Spinal cord transection at the level of T4 results in loss of sensation and motor control below T4, as well as incontinence, hyperreflexia, and extensor plantar responses.

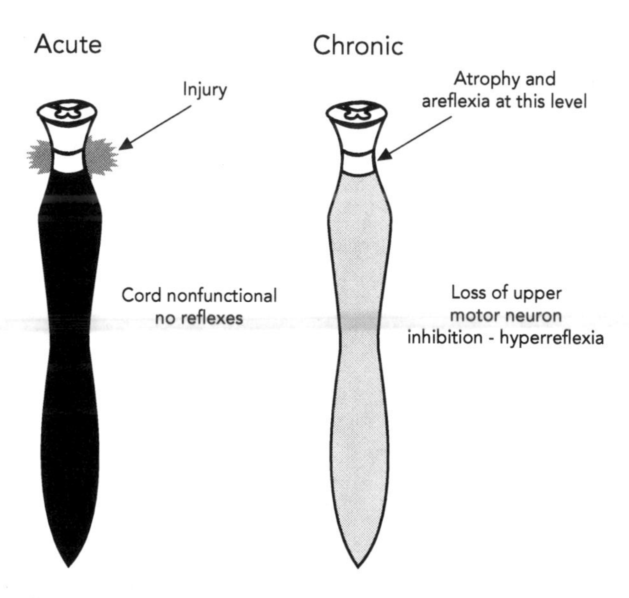

Figure 2.54 Spinal cord shock manifests 6 weeks to 8 weeks following a spinal injury, and is characterized by a total loss of all spinal cord function below the level of the spinal cord lesion. During this time period, every segment of the cord acts as though it were injured, and reflexes below the level of the lesion are lost.

- Etiologies:
  - Trauma
  - Transverse myelitis (usually postinfectious or demyelinative)
  - Tumor
  - Radiation injury

Note: Spinal cord shock (see Figure 2.54).

With any cord injury of significance, there is a 6-week to 8-week period of spinal shock characterized by a total loss of all spinal cord function below the lesion, as though every segment of the cord were injured directly. During this time period, the reflexes are lost.

2. Hemisection/Brown-Séquard Syndrome

- Clinical features:
  - Contralateral loss of pain and temperature beginning one level to two levels below the lesion caused by damage to the anterolateral systems (spinothalamic tracts) (Figure 2.55).

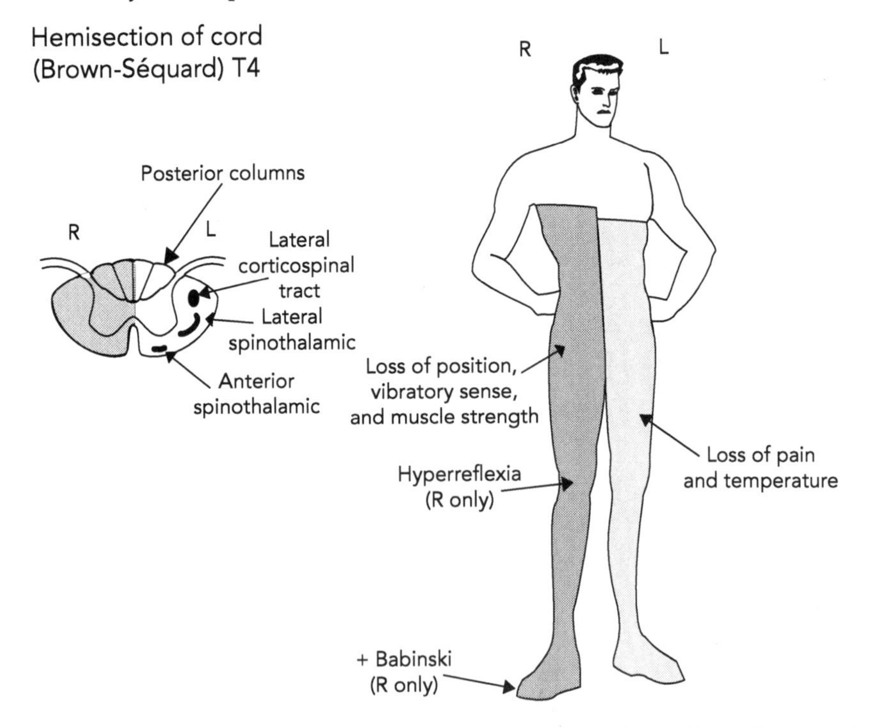

Figure 2.55 Right T4 Brown-Séquard syndrome: contralateral loss of pain and temperature one level to two levels below T4 (spinothalamic tract); ipsilateral loss of position and vibratory sensation below T4 (posterior columns); ipsilateral motor paralysis below T4 (corticospinal tract).

- Ipsilateral loss of position and vibratory sensation below the level of the lesion, caused by damage to the posterior columns (fasciculus gracilis [from lower extremity] and cuneatus [from upper extremity]).
- Ipsilateral motor paralysis below the level of the lesion, caused by damage to the lateral corticospinal tract.
- *Sparing* of light touch.

▪ Etiologies:
- Trauma
- Compression from abscess, hematoma, or neoplasm
- Multiple sclerosis

3. Syringomyelia

Syringomyelia (Figure 2.56) involves formation of a syrinx, or cyst, in the central gray matter of the spinal cord.

▪ Clinical features:
- Loss of pain and temperature sensations *below* the level of the lesion caused by damage to crossing spinothalamic fibers in the anterior

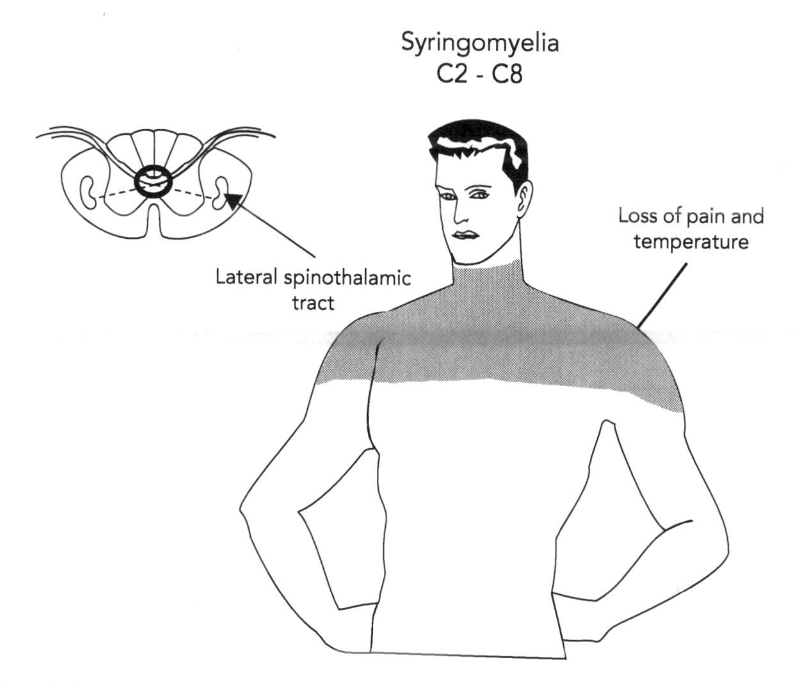

Figure 2.56 Syringomyelia leads to loss of pain and temperature sensations, initially involving the proximal shoulders in a cape distribution.

commissure. There is preserved vibratory and position sense mediated by the dorsal columns; hence, this is a dissociative sensory loss.
- As lesion enlarges, weakness and atrophy develop.
- Damage to anterior horn cells eventually causes LMN deficits at the level of the lesion.
- Damage to corticospinal tracts may ultimately lead to UMN signs.
- Possible late involvement may involve the posterior columns, leading to loss of position and vibratory sense.
- These typically are cervical and lead to sensory symptoms over the shoulders, known as a cape-like distribution as in Batman's or Superman's cape.

■ Etiologies:
- Chiari I malformation (characterized by displaced cerebellar tonsils downward through the foramen magnum, usually a congenital malformation)
- Tumor of spinal cord
- Hemorrhage
- Trauma

4. Anterior Spinal Artery Syndrome

■ Vascular review:
- The anterior spinal artery supplies blood to the anterior two-thirds of the spinal cord (Figure 2.57).
- The anterior spinal artery receives blood from smaller medullary arteries at irregular intervals.
- Pressure in the anterior spinal artery is lower than normal arterial pressure.

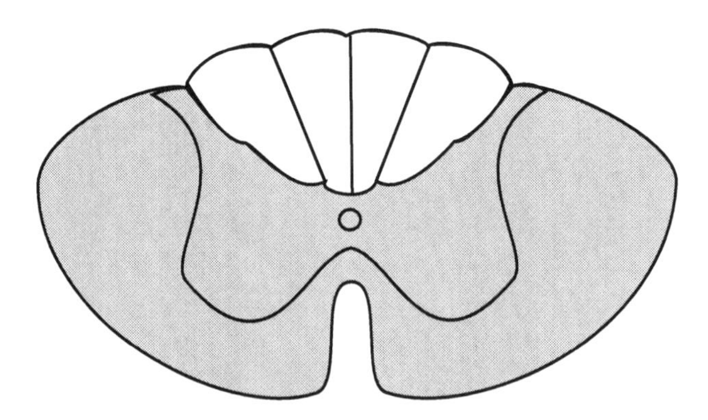

Figure 2.57 The anterior spinal artery supplies blood to the anterior two-thirds of the spinal cord, as shown in gray.

- Blood supply to the anterior spinal artery is tenuous in two regions (Figure 2.58):
  (1) T1 to T4
  (2) T10 to L3: an area dependent on perfusion from one large artery that is a branch off the aorta, the artery of Adamkiewicz
- There are no vascular anastomoses within the substance of the normal spinal cord.

■ Clinical features of anterior spinal artery syndrome:

- Loss of muscle strength below the level of the lesion caused by damage to the anterior horn cells
- Bilateral loss of pain and temperature sensations 1 to 2 levels below the lesion caused by damage to the anterolateral pathways (i.e., spinothalamic tracts)
- Sparing of dorsal column functions (position and vibratory senses)

■ Etiologies:

- Dissecting aortic aneurysm may shear off origin of an important spinal artery

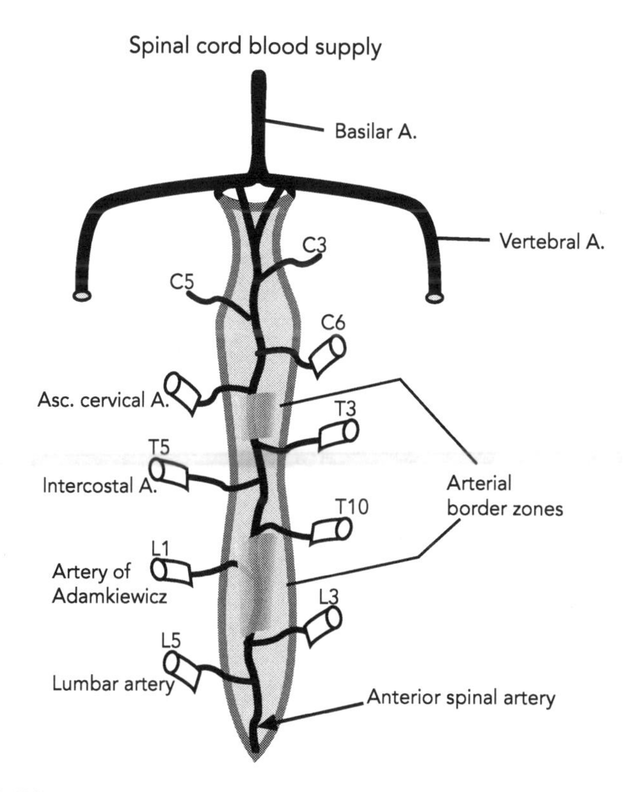

Figure 2.58 Segments T1 to T4 and T10 to L3 are poorly vascularized and are especially at risk for ischemic injury.

- Hypotensive crisis
- Cardiac surgery with prolonged cross-clamping of aorta
- Atherosclerosis of aorta at origin of an important feeding artery
- Emboli
- AVM (arteriovenous malformation) of cord with shunting of blood from the cord

5. Tabetic Syndrome

Disease processes may specifically affect the larger posterior fibers of the dorsal (posterior) roots that are destined to become the posterior columns (Figure 2.59).

- Clinical features:
  - Loss of vibratory and position sensations below the level of the lesion
    (1) Usually symmetrical
    (2) Predominantly involving the lower extremities
    (3) Leads to a sensory ataxia due to loss of position sense
  - Associated loss of deep pain or touch sensations in long-standing cases
  - Areflexia—due to loss of the afferent limb of the reflex arc (Figure 2.60)
  - Hypotonia—loss of proprioceptors from muscle spindles, thus eliminating feedback to maintain proper tone
  - Bladder dysfunction
  - Lightning pains

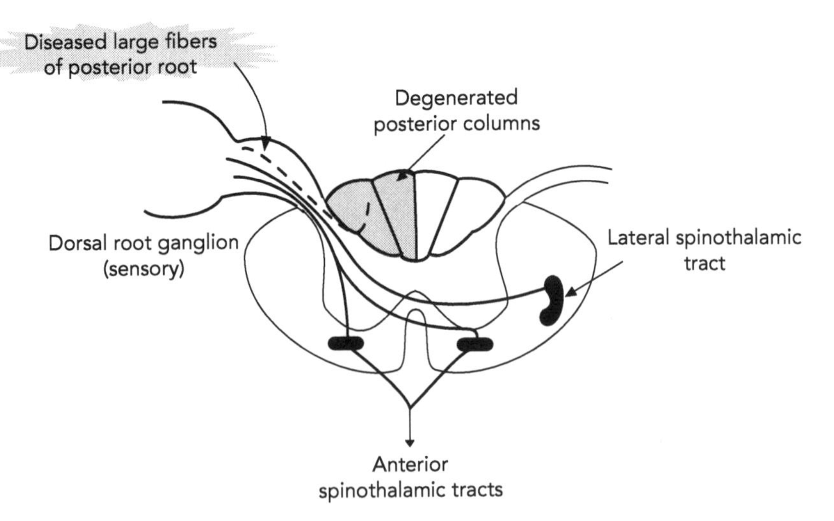

Figure 2.59 Tabetic syndrome (dorsal column syndrome). Gray area shows distribution of pathology, typically involving dorsal columns as well as dorsal roots and ganglia.

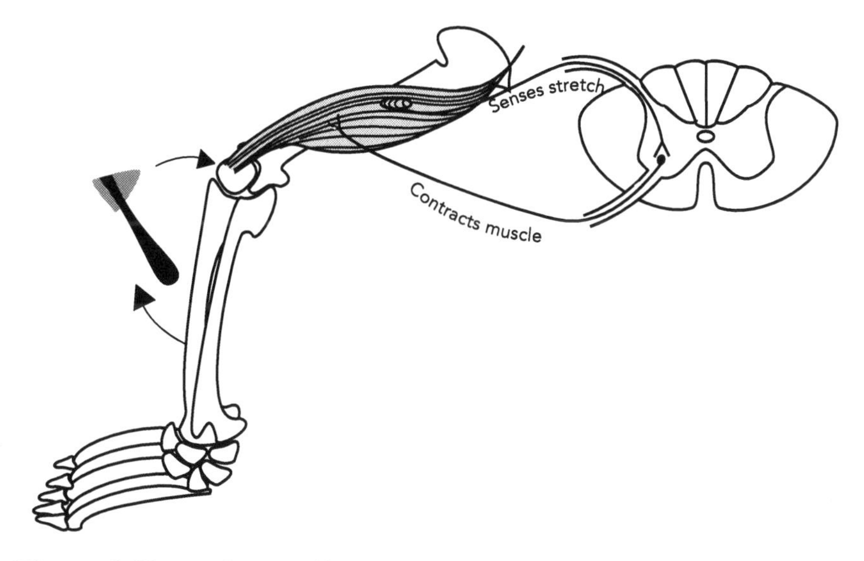

Figure 2.60 Areflexia and hypotonia result from a loss of afferent information from muscle spindles, thus eliminating feedback to maintain proper muscle tone.

- Etiologies:
  - Tabes dorsalis—one form of tertiary neurosyphilis
  - Diabetes mellitus

6. Combined Systems Degeneration

This syndrome is caused by disease processes that directly affect the posterior columns and lateral corticospinal tracts (Figure 2.61). This may be difficult

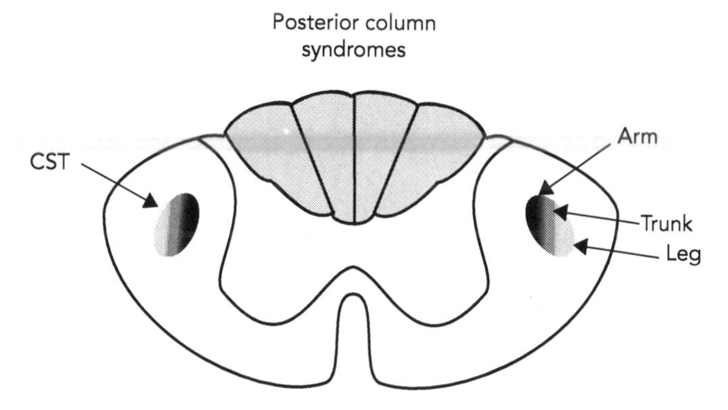

Figure 2.61 Distribution of pathology in subacute combined degeneration of the spinal cord.

to distinguish from tabes dorsalis due to the common posterior column involvement.

- Vitamin B_{12} deficiency:
  - Diffuse involvement of dorsal columns and lateral corticospinal tracts
  - Loss of position and vibratory sensations below the level of the lesion
  - Loss of motor function below the level of the lesion
  - Less common cause is copper deficiency: hypocupremic myelopathy
  - B_{12} deficiency can also affect other areas of the nervous system: cerebral hemisphere, optic nerve, cerebellum, peripheral nerve
- Motor neuron disease—amyotrophic lateral sclerosis (ALS):
  - Involvement of corticospinal tracts and anterior horn cells
  - Combination of UMN (corticospinal tracts) and LMN (anterior horn cell) signs
  - Also known as Lou Gehrig's disease

3

The Peripheral Nervous System: Nerves and Muscles

A. ROOTS AND NERVES: MAKING THE CONNECTIONS

1. Function of Peripheral Nerves

- Relay sensory information to spinal cord
- Carry motor innervation to muscle

2. Cardinal Signs of Peripheral Nerve Disease

Output of lower motor neuron (anterior horn cell) blocked

- Weakness
- Wasting
- Areflexia

Various patterns of sensory loss

- Nerve root disease—dermatomal pattern
- Mononeuropathy—follows innervation of peripheral nerve
- Polyneuropathy—distal greater than proximal (i.e., stocking-glove pattern)

Sidebar: Polyneuropathy is often related to nutritional factors in the peripheral nerve axonal metabolic transport systems; thus, the most distal portions of the nerve are affected first. Symptoms in the hands are not usually seen until there is involvement in the lower extremities up to the knees.

Variable autonomic involvement examples: diabetes, amyloidosis

3. Anatomical Organization of PNS (Peripheral Nervous System)

- Nerve roots (radicular portion of nerves)—from spinal cord through the intervertebral foramina
- Plexus—area of mixing of nerve roots to ultimately form the peripheral nerves
- Peripheral nerves

B. RADICULAR NERVE INVOLVEMENT (THE ROOTS)

1. Dorsal Root and Dorsal Root Ganglia Disease

Anatomical considerations

- Loss of sensory information to the spinal cord and the brain
- Large fibers affected first (mediating position and vibration perception)

Clinical picture

- Unable to feel where feet are—slapping gait
- Difficulty walking in the dark (loss of visual cues)
- Bladder may become involved—impaired sense of detrusor muscle stretching leads to hypotonic, flaccid bladder
- Difficult to distinguish from posterior column disease

Etiologies

- Tabes dorsalis
- Diabetes mellitus

Note: Herpes zoster virus may lie dormant in the dorsal root ganglia for years. With reactivation there is painful herpetic eruption (blisters) in the corresponding sensory dermatome.

2. Nerve Root Disease

Anatomical considerations

- May be compressed in subarachnoid space by protruding disc (nucleus pulposus).
- C5 through C7 and L4 through S1 are areas of greatest instability (Figure 3.1).
- The lateral ligaments supporting the cord are relatively weak; thus, disc herniations most frequently occur laterally.
- Posteriorly displaced discs may compress multiple nerve roots and result in bilateral rather than unilateral symptoms. This is particularly true at the level of the cauda equina below the bottom of the spinal cord.
- Most lumbar slipped discs occur at the vertebral interspaces L4, L5 or L5 through S1. Because the nerve root has already exited below the higher vertebral body, the disc will compress the descending root from the lower level. Thus, a classic L4, L5 central disc herniation will cause an L5 radiculopathy. By the same token, a lateral L5 through S1 radiculopathy will cause an S1 radiculopathy (Figure 3.2).

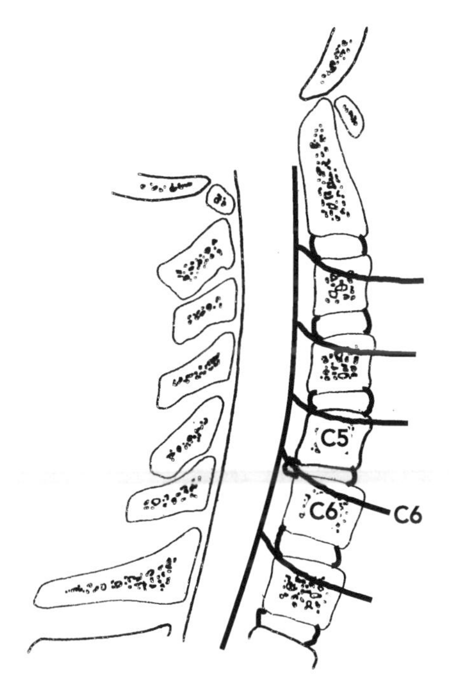

Figure 3.1 C5-C6 herniated disc compressing the C6 nerve root. There is relatively little space for the cord at this cervical level, and a larger disc could compress the spinal cord itself. C1-C7 nerve roots exist above their vertebral bodies, C8 nerve root exists at the C7-T1 vertebral level, and the nerve roots in the thoracic region exit below their named vertebral bodies.

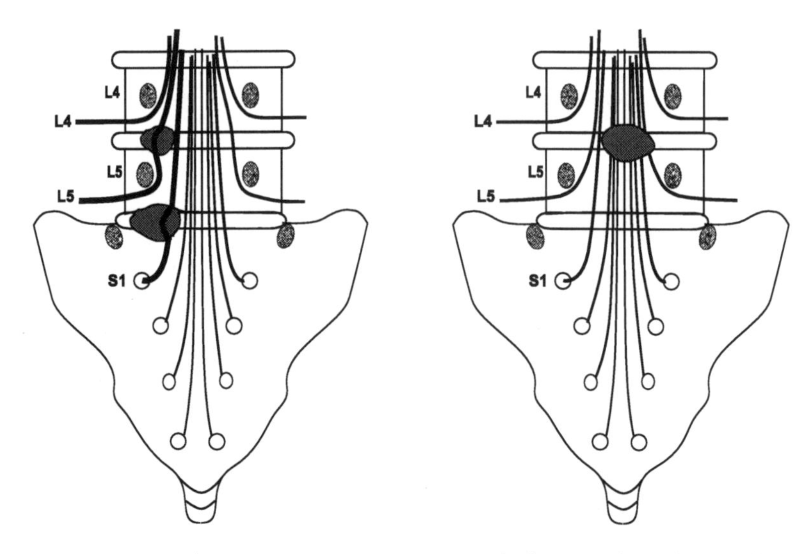

Figure 3.2 Relationships between herniated discs and lumbosacral nerve roots. Left: The laterally herniated L4-L5 disc compresses the L5 root, and L5-S1 disc compresses the S1 nerve root. Right: A central disc herniation at level L4-5 asymmetrically compresses the L5 nerve root and multiple descending sacral nerve roots below.

Clinical features

- Motor loss in muscles innervated by that cord segment:
  - Wasting (loss of muscle bulk = atrophy)
  - Areflexia (if cord segment is involved in a motor reflex)
    - Dermatomal sensory change as radiating pain, paresthesias (pins and needles), or anesthesia (Figure 3.3)
    - Neck or low back pain
    - If the herniation compresses the spinal cord itself (as may occur in the cervical or thoracic region), then long tract (UMN [upper motor neurons]) signs may be seen below the level of the lesion.

Lesions causing root entrapment

- Arachnoiditis
- Carcinoma, metastases
- Meningitis

Diseases with propensity toward root involvement

- Guillain-Barré syndrome (acute inflammatory demyelinating polyradiculoneuropathy):
  - Acute inflammatory demyelinating polyradiculoneuropathy
  - Postinfectious, postvaccine, postsurgical

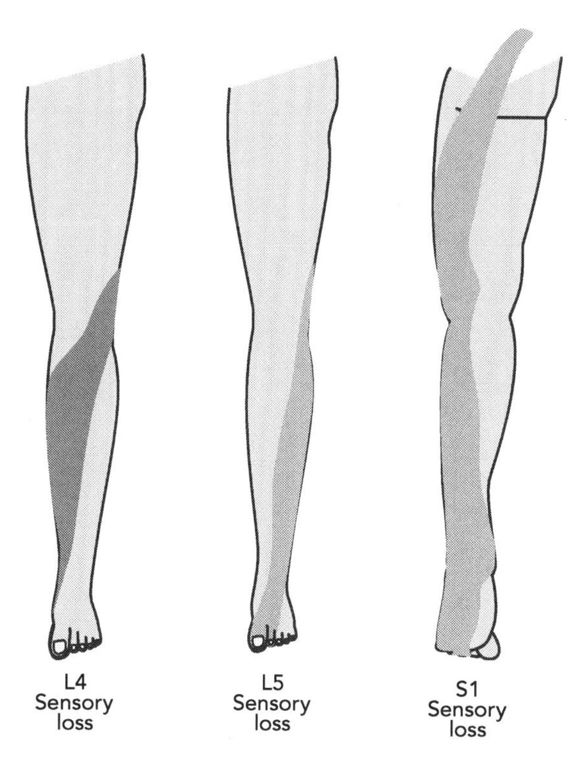

Figure 3.3 Distribution of sensory loss for L4, L5, and S1 radiculopathies.

- Classic type presents with an ascending paralysis from feet and legs up to the arms and intercostal muscles affecting respiration
- CSF (cerebrospinal fluid) cytoalbuminologic dissociation (low cells, high protein)
- No significant sensory loss
- Gradual fairly complete recovery is the rule

- CIDP (chronic inflammatory demyelinating polyneuropathy):
  - Chronic version of Guillain-Barré without complete recovery
  - Higher CSF protein levels than in Guillain-Barré

C. THE PLEXI

1. Brachial Plexus (Figure 3.4)

Anterior primary rami lesions

- Rhomboid, serratus anterior weakness
- Segmental weakness

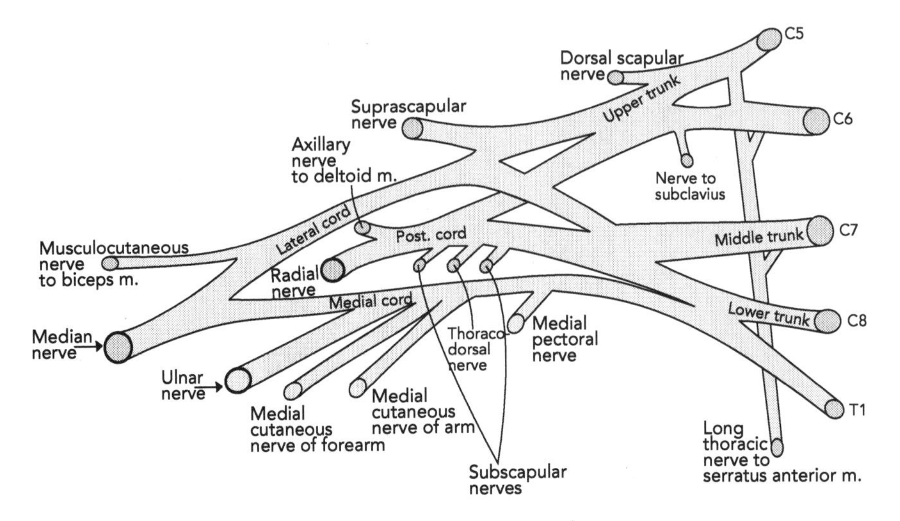

Figure 3.4 The brachial plexus.

- Involvement of T1 associated with Horner syndrome—due to proximity of the sympathetic outflow track, ultimately providing innervation to the ipsilateral pupil and eyelid, and producing, when lesioned, the deficits of a small pupil (i.e., miosis, and a droopy eyelid, ptosis)

Upper trunk lesions (C5, C6)—associated with Erb's palsy (congenital brachial plexus palsy, usually associated with fetal shoulder dystocia)

- Weakness of supraspinatus, infraspinatus, deltoid, biceps, and supinator muscles
- Arm hangs limply at side, medially rotated and pronated (waiter's tip posture)

Lower plexus injuries (C7, C8, T1)—Klumpke's palsy (complete congenital brachial plexus palsy)

- Weakness of intrinsic muscles of hand including finger flexors

Radiation fibrosis entrapping brachial plexus

- Particularly postbreast cancer radiation

Infiltration of the plexus by tumor

- Very painful

Brachial neuritis

- Viral/postviral syndrome
- Resolves spontaneously

Cervical rib

- Traction on lower trunk of brachial plexus (C8, T1) as it is stretched over cervical rib
- Interosseus muscle weakness
- Ulnar distribution sensory loss
- May be confused clinically with ulnar neuropathy

2. The Lumbosacral Plexus (Figure 3.5)

Pathology usually due to compression

- Tumor (typically primary of uterus, bladder, prostate, colon, or lymph glands)
- Metastases
- Gravid uterus

Clinical features

- Back pain
- Patchy sensory loss
- Patchy, flaccid, areflexic motor loss with a mixed picture of nerve root and peripheral nerve patterns
- Variable bladder and bowel involvement

Note: It may be very difficult to distinguish *bilateral lumbosacral plexus* disease from *cauda equina* lesions. Both lead to asymmetrical lower extremity motor and sensory deficits with pain. In contrast, *conus medullaris* lesions cause bilaterally symmetrical deficits with early urinary or fecal incontinence.

3. Peripheral Nerves (the Branches)

Polyneuropathy

- Anatomical considerations:
  - Symmetric polyneuropathy
  - Multifocal, mononeuritis multiplex
  - Isolated nerve

- Pathophysiology:
  - Axonal
    - Loss of axonal integrity and ability to transport nutrients down the axon
    - The longest and most distal portions of the nerves are earliest and most affected; hence, stocking-glove distribution of weakness and numbness. Examples of etiologies: diabetes, uremia, alcohol, vitamin B_{12} deficiency, hypothyroidism

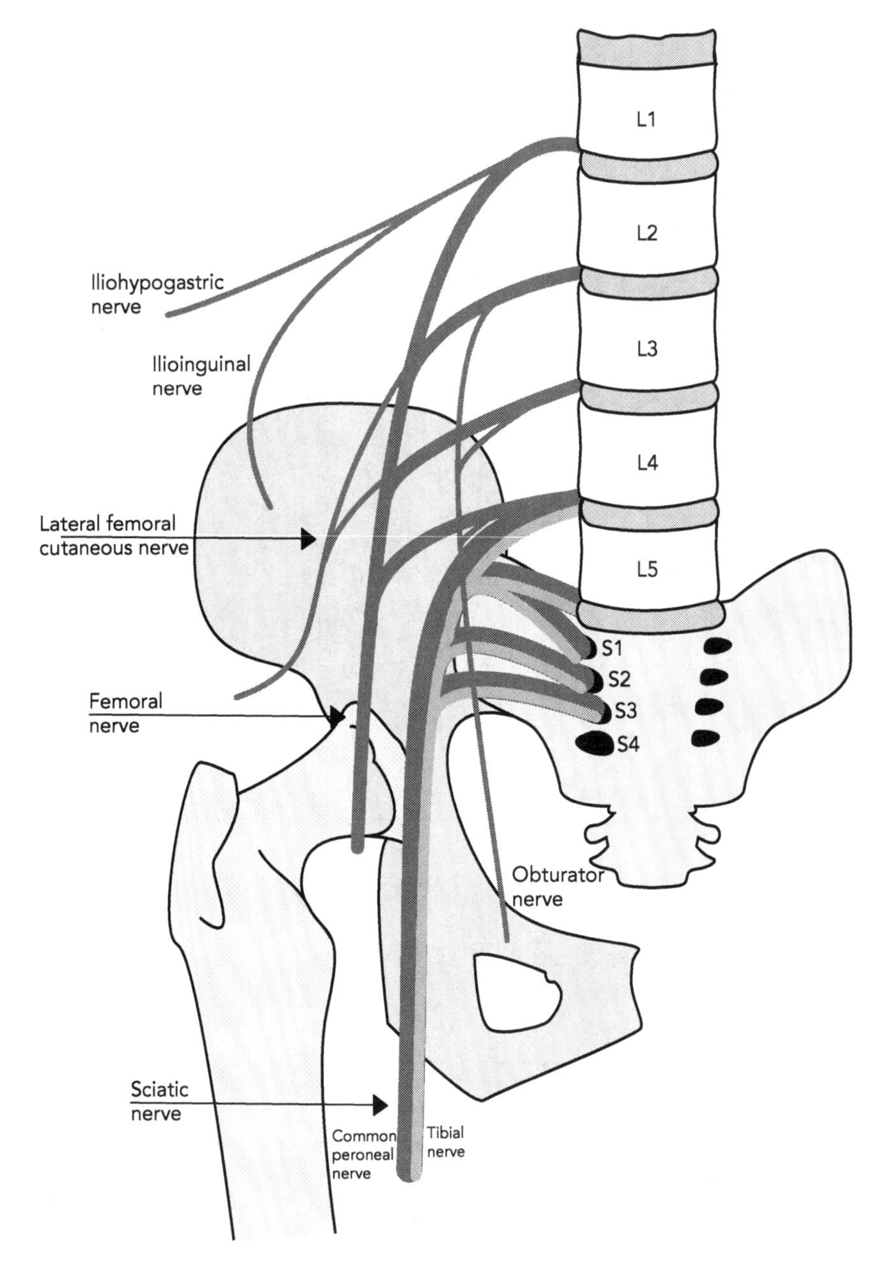

Figure 3.5 The lumbosacral plexus.

- Demyelinative
  - Segmental demyelination
  - Etiologies: Guillain-Barré syndrome, diphtheria, lead poisoning
  - Clinical features: legs affected first (exception: lead neuropathy where the arms and legs are involved similarly)

Mononeuropathy

- Etiology:
  - Compressive
  - Traumatic
  - Underlying disease (diabetes, Behçet disease, collagen vascular disease, sarcoidosis, monoclonal gammopathy)
    - A person with preexisting symmetric polyneuropathy is more subject to compressive neuropathy.

- Common syndromes:
  - Radial nerve palsy
  - Median nerve palsy
  - Ulnar neuropathy
  - Intercostal neuralgia
  - Lateral femoral cutaneous nerve palsy (meralgia paresthetica)
  - Femoral neuropathy
  - Sciatic neuropathy
  - Peroneal nerve palsy

- Radial nerve palsy:
  - Mechanism: compression of radial nerve in spiral groove of humerus

  - Etiology
    - Falling asleep with arm over back of bar chair (Saturday night palsy) or paramour (bridegroom palsy)
    - Fracture of humerus

  - Clinical presentation
    - Absent triceps function
    - Wrist drop (w*R*ist drop is due to *R*adial nerve palsy)
    - Anesthesia of dorsum of hand between thumb and index finger (Figure 3.6)

  - Treatment
    - Splint wrist in extension
    - Physical therapy to prevent contractures of fingers
    - Time

- Median nerve palsy (carpal tunnel syndrome [CTS]):
  - Mechanism: compression of median nerve as it passes under the flexor retinaculum of the wrist

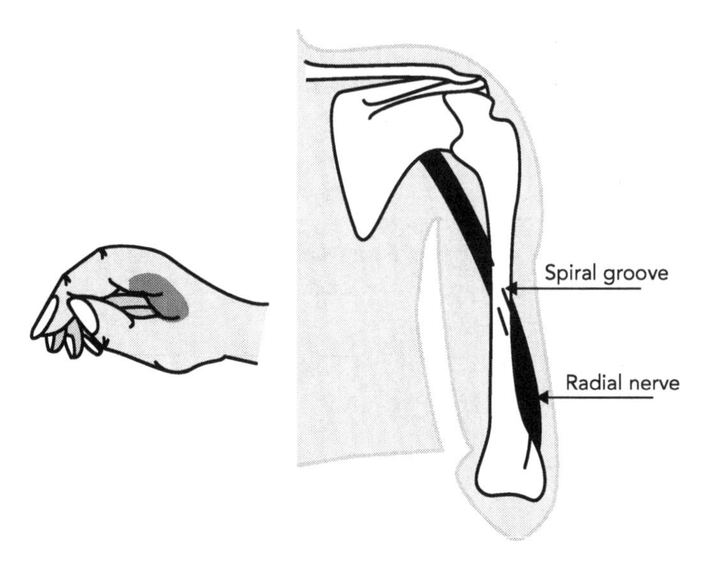

Figure 3.6 Radial nerve palsy.

- Etiology
  - Diabetes
  - Hypothyroidism
  - Acromegaly
  - Amyloidosis
  - Pregnancy
  - Lupus
  - Idiopathic
- Clinical presentation
  - Tingling in palm of hand in median sensory distribution, particularly at night (Figure 3.7)
  - Later—weakness of apposition of thumb and finger flexors (weak grip)
  - Atrophy of thenar eminence (later)
  - Positive Tinel's sign (tingling of hand upon volar wrist tap)
  - Nerve conduction study shows absent median nerve sensory potential and prolonged distal motor nerve conduction latency
- Treatment: splint to straighten wrist at night
  - Prescribe for underlying problem
  - Anti-inflammatory medicines, steroid injections
  - Surgical release of nerve within the carpal tunnel

■ Ulnar neuropathy:

- Mechanism: compression of ulnar nerve as it passes behind the medial epicondyle of the humerus
- Etiology: leaning on elbows

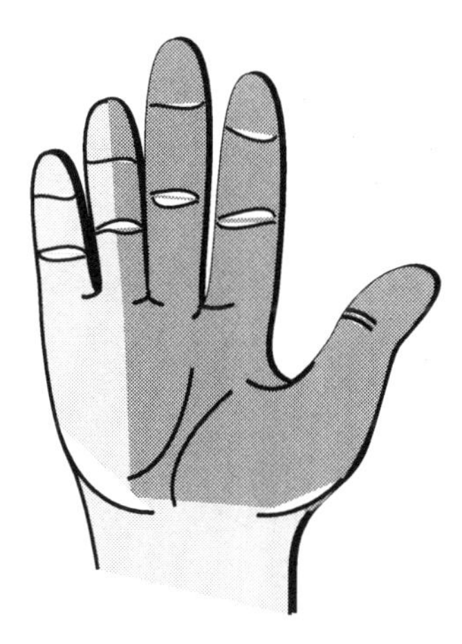

Figure 3.7 Shaded area shows distribution of involved median nerve innervation in carpal tunnel syndrome (CTS). Typically, the sensory symptoms are limited to the fingers. Motor weakness and muscle atrophy may also involve the more proximal palmar region.

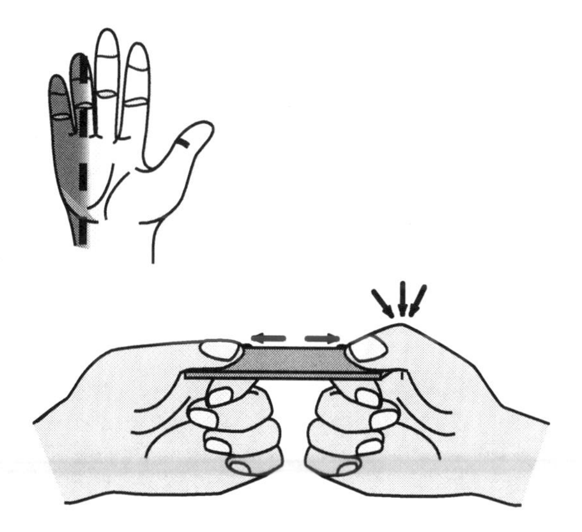

Figure 3.8 Positive Froment's sign, where the interphalangeal joint rises to compensate for weakness of thumb adduction in ulnar neuropathy. Sensory distribution is shown in the top portion.

- Clinical presentation
  - Tingling medial aspect of hand (pinky and half of the ring finger)
  - Weakness of interossei and hypothenar eminence
  - Positive Froment's sign (Figure 3.8)
  - Ulnar nerve conduction velocity slowed at elbow on electrophysiological testing

- Treatment: stop exacerbating behavior
  - Prescribe for any underlying metabolic disorder
  - Nerve transposition procedure (moves the nerve to avoid area of compression or entrapment)

■ Intercostal neuralgia:

- Clinical presentation: band-like dysesthetic sensation in dermatomal distribution around trunk
- Etiology
  - Diabetes
  - Note: spinal cord lesions due to masses or multiple sclerosis may also produce band-like sensory loss.
  - Treatment: treat the underlying problem.

■ Lateral femoral cutaneous nerve palsy (meralgia paresthetica):

- Mechanism: lateral femoral cutaneous nerve arises from L2, L3 and reaches leg by passing under the inguinal ligament where it may be entrapped.
- Etiology
  - Diabetes
  - Pregnancy
  - Ascites
  - Rapid weight loss/gain
  - Idiopathic
- Clinical feature: irritating dysesthesias/anesthesia over anterolateral thigh

■ Femoral neuropathy:

- Mechanism: nerve arises from L2 through L4, passes through body of psoas muscle under inguinal ligament to anterior compartment of thigh, and may be compressed in retroperitoneal space (Figure 3.9).
- Clinical features
  - Weakness of hip flexion and knee extension
  - Sensory loss of anterior and medial thigh and medial leg and foot (saphenous nerve)
- Etiology
  - Spontaneous hemorrhage into body of psoas muscle, especially in patients on anticoagulants
  - Retroperitoneal tumor
  - Diabetes

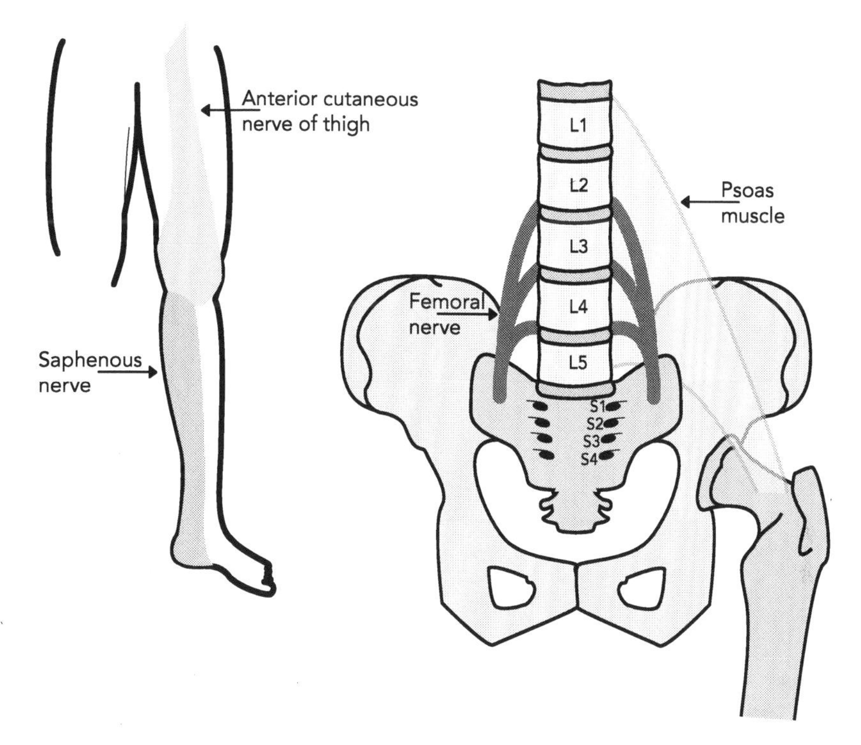

Figure 3.9 Femoral nerve arises from L2 through L4. Left portion shows sensory innervation of femoral nerve.

- Treatment: reverse any clotting abnormalities
  - Remove hematoma if present
  - Treat underlying disease
  - Physical therapy to strengthen femoral innervated muscles

■ Sciatic neuropathy:

- Mechanism: arises from L4, L5, and S1 through S3, exits pelvis through greater sciatic foramen, passes through posterior thigh, and at popliteal fossa divides into tibial and common peroneal nerves
- Etiology: poorly placed IM (intramuscular) injection
  - Trauma, including IM injections (important to aim for upper outer quadrant of buttock to avoid sciatic nerve)
  - Infarction of nerve trunk—diabetes, polyarteritis nodosa
- Clinical presentation: weakness of dorsiflexion and plantar flexion, eversion and inversion of foot
  - Weak knee flexors
  - Sensory loss below the knee sparing medial aspect of the leg and ankle

- L5 radiculopathy may simulate sciatic nerve lesion (Figure 3.10 shows sensory difference), and EMG (electromyogram) or imaging may be needed to distinguish these

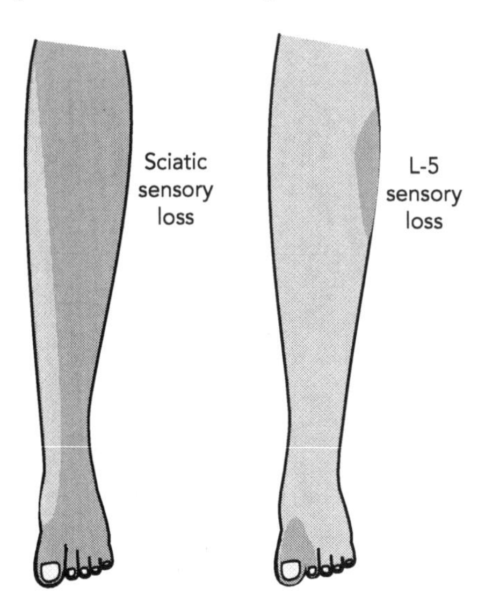

Figure 3.10 The more extensive sensory loss in a sciatic nerve lesion helps to differentiate this from an L5 root lesion.

- Treatment
  - Time
  - Physical therapy

- Peroneal nerve palsy:
  - Mechanism: compression of peroneal nerve against the head of the fibula at the knee
  - Clinical presentation: foot drop
    - Weak everters of foot
    - Inconsistent sensory loss over lateral aspect of leg and dorsum of foot
  - Etiology: prolonged and frequent leg crossing
    - Trauma
    - Underlying disease (diabetes)
  - Treatment: remove risk factors if possible
    - Splint to straighten the dropped foot
    - Physical therapy

4

Special Applications of Neuro-Logic: Neurologic Classics

A. COMA

1. Definition

Coma is defined as the absence of awareness of one's self and one's environment. More specifically, it can be described as an unarousable and unresponsive state in which the patient remains with eyes closed. On neurological examination, the comatose patient has no purposeful response to nociceptive (i.e., painful) stimulation.

Localization of *coma*: coma is caused by lesions in two locations:

- *Bihemispheric*
- *Brainstem*

A gray zone of *altered states* exists between coma and consciousness (*vide infra*).

2. Consciousness

Definition

Consciousness is the awareness of one's self and one's environment. Conscious behavior is determined by arousal and content.

One might think that coma is simply an alteration in arousal; however, content is included in the definition because continuous eye-closed coma almost never persists beyond 4 weeks. Coma is then replaced by sleep–wakefulness cycles. Thus, the severely brain-injured patient may appear awake (*arousal intact*) but is totally unresponsive (*no content*). This is known as a persistent vegetative state.

Maintenance of consciousness

Consciousness is maintained by diffuse cortical and limbic projections of the ascending reticular activating system (RAS) (Figure 4.1). All sensory systems synapse on the brainstem RAS. The cerebral cortex is kept awake via RAS–cortical projections. Control of the level of consciousness can be said to revolve around three pertinent aspects:

- Alertness—depends on mesencephalic reticular formation, thalamus, and cortex
- Attention—depends on the same, as well as frontoparietal association cortex
- Awareness—depends on our ability to combine various higher order forms of sensory, motor, emotional, and mnemonic information from different brain regions into a unified content

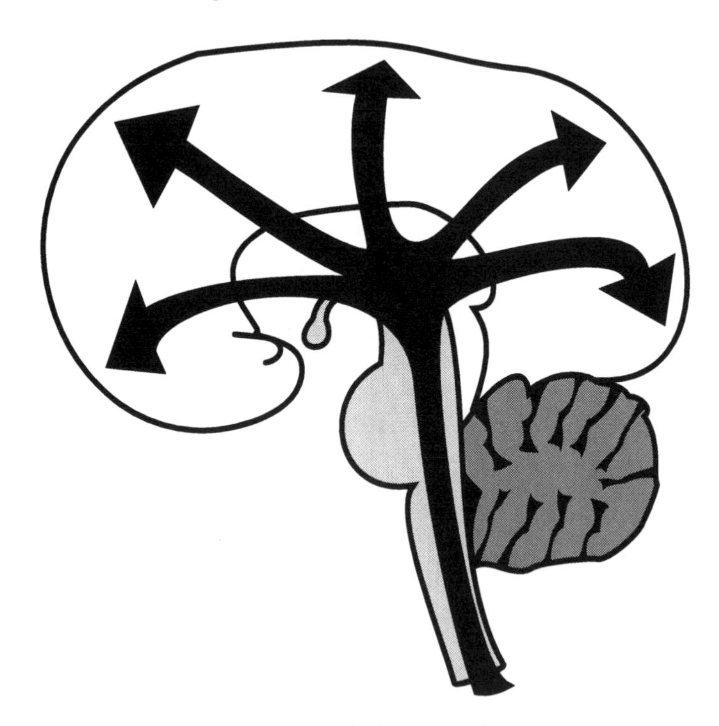

Figure 4.1 Diffuse projections of the reticular activating system (RAS) maintaining consciousness.

Coma etiologies

- Bilateral cortical disease may result from:
  - Metabolic derangements
    - Hypoxia
    - Hypo/Hyperglycemia
    - Hypo/Hypernatremia
    - Hypercalcemia
    - Hypothyroidism
    - Hepatic encephalopathy
    - Thiamine deficiency
    - High fever
  - Intoxications
    - ETOH (ethanol or ethyl alcohol)
    - Barbiturates
    - Tranquilizers
    - Tricyclic antidepressants
    - Other sedative hypnotics
  - Diffuse infiltrative processes
    - Meningoencephalitis
    - Gliomatosis cerebri
  - Other

    Subarachnoid hemorrhage

    All of the above processes may affect brainstem function as well.

- Brainstem dysfunction may also result from:
  - Supratentorial mass lesions with herniation
  - Cerebellar mass lesions with brainstem compression
  - Cerebellar tonsillar herniation
  - Intrinsic brainstem disease
    - Pontine hemorrhage
    - Brainstem vascular insufficiency (stroke)
    - Brainstem glioma

- Herniation:

  Displacement of brain tissue from one compartment to another

The cranial vault is a fixed space housing the brain, blood, and CSF (cerebrospinal fluid). As a mass develops, the brain becomes compressed and the extracellular fluid and blood are squeezed out. This in turn causes a compensatory decrease in CSF production. If a mass continues to enlarge, intracranial pressure increases and vector pressure forces develop:

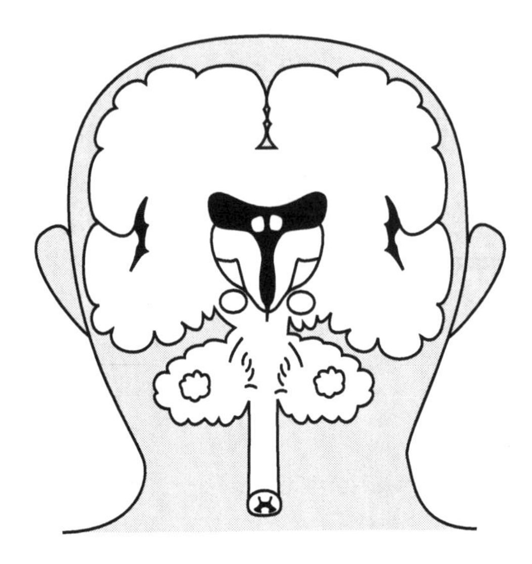

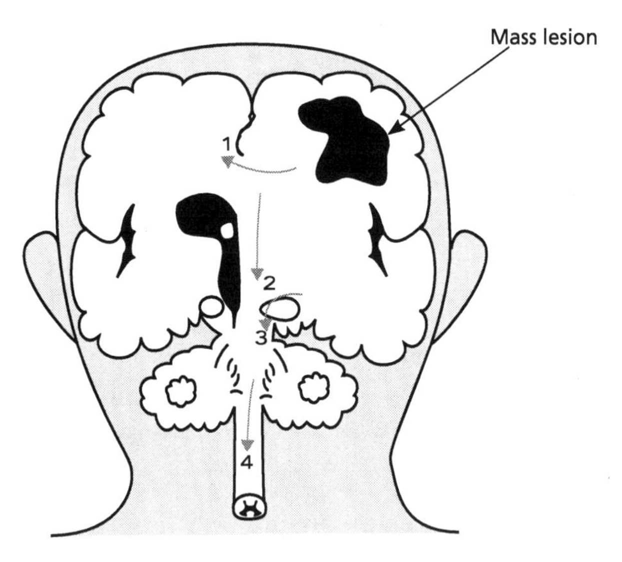

Figure 4.2 Direction of herniation shown from upper figure (normal) to lower figure (1, subfalcine; 2, transtentorial diencephalic; 3, uncal; and 4, cerebellar).

- Types of herniations (Figure 4.2):
  - Subfalcine: cingulate gyrus herniates under the falx cerebri
    Symptom:
    - contralateral leg weakness
  - Transtentorial diencephalic: the edematous hemispheres bilaterally exert downward pressure onto the diencephalon (i.e., thalamus) that may then be transmitted into the brainstem.

Symptoms:
- Depression of consciousness and typically bilateral progressive brainstem dysfunction

- Uncal: medial temporal lobe herniates under tentorium cerebelli
  Symptoms:
  - Dilatation of ipsilateral pupil and progressive CN (cranial nerve) III palsy
  - Occipital lobe infarction manifested by visual problems, such as cortical blindness
  - Depression of level of consciousness
  - Ipsilateral hemiparesis—a false localizing sign, due to the force of the uncal herniation pushing against the upper brainstem and forcing the opposite cerebral peduncle into the edge of the tentorium cerebelli. For example, a LEFT uncal herniation will result in notching of the RIGHT cerebral peduncle, carrying RIGHT corticospinal tract fibers to the left side of the body, thus creating hemiparisis ipsilateral to the side of the uncal herniation. Compression of the lateral corticospinal tracts opposite the herniation on the edge of the tentorium cerebelli, known as Kernohan's notch (Figure 4.3)
- Cerebellar tonsillar herniation downward through the foramen magnum
  Symptoms:
  - Medullary compression with rapid cardiorespiratory arrest

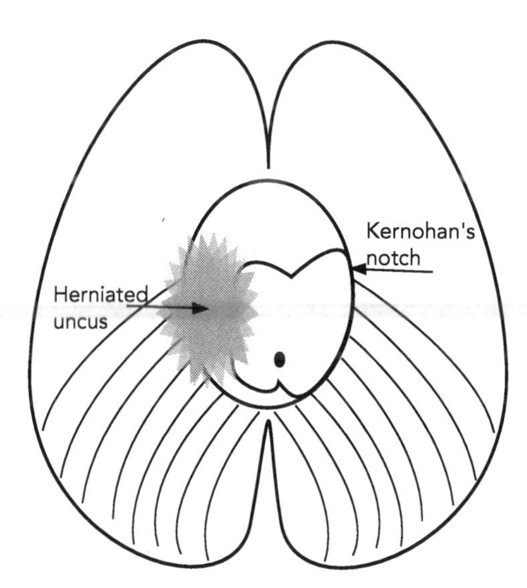

Figure 4.3 LEFT uncal herniation results in downward and lateral compression of the brainstem forcing the contralateral cerebral peduncle into the edge of the tentorium cerebelli, creating Kernohan's notch. This disrupts RIGHT corticospinal tract fibers and results in a hemiparesis ipsilateral to the side of the uncal herniation.

Examination of the comatose patient

- Check vital signs—for signs of increased intracranial pressure (ICP):
  - Bradycardia
  - Widened pulse pressure [increased systolic BP (blood pressure), decreased diastolic BP]
  - Respiratory change (see respiratory patterns following). This triad is denoted as the Cushing reflex.
- Assess level of consciousness:
  - Clouding of consciousness—a state of reduced wakefulness or awareness that includes excitability and irritability alternating with drowsiness. More advanced clouding produces a confusional state in which stimuli are more consistently misinterpreted.
  - Delirium—a more florid state characterized by disorientation, fear, irritability, misperception of sensory stimuli, and often visual hallucinations. Delirium implies fluctuating levels of consciousness.
  - Stupor—unresponsiveness from which the subject can be only partially aroused with vigorous and repeated stimuli
  - Coma—unarousable unresponsiveness
- Respiratory patterns (Figure 4.4):
  - Hemispheric coma: Cheyne-Stokes respirations—a crescendo–decrescendo pattern of hyperpnea alternating regularly with apnea. The localization is due to bihemispheric coma and this may be due to

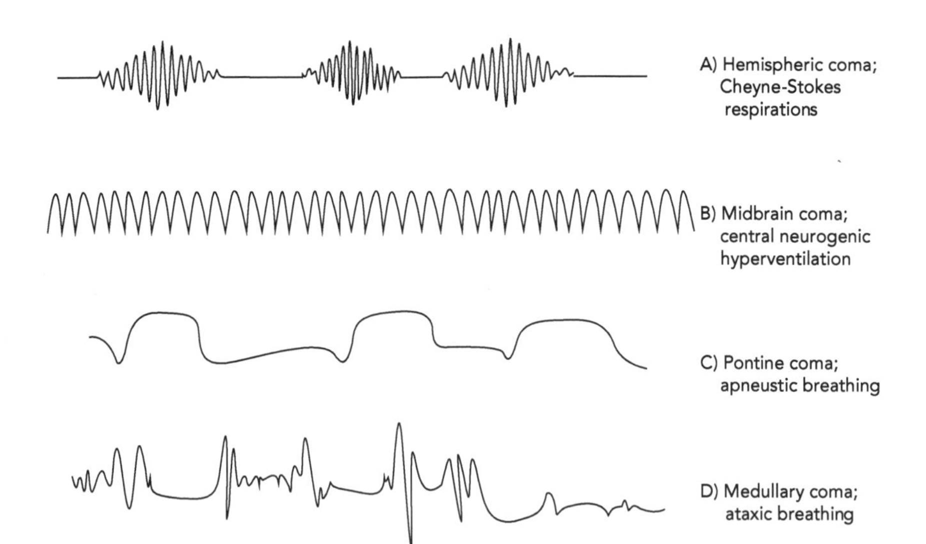

Figure 4.4 Respiratory patterns in coma associated with lesions at specific levels.

metabolic brain dysfunction as well as bilateral deep-seated cerebral lesions.

- Midbrain coma: central neurogenic hyperventilation—sustained regular deep hyperpnea. Localization is brainstem tegmentum, usually low midbrain to the middle third of the pons.
- Pontine coma: apneustic breathing—prolonged inspiratory cramp. Rarely seen but if present implies damage to the respiratory control mechanisms located at the mid- or caudal-pontine level. Clinically this is mainly seen with pontine infarction.
- Medullary coma: ataxic breathing—completely irregular and uncoordinated breathing pattern, due to involvement of respiratory centers in the reticular formation of the dorsomedial part of the medulla.

■ Pupils (Figure 4.5):

- Hemispheric coma: pupils are midposition in size and normal. The sympathetic and parasympathetic fibers that dilate and constrict the pupil are below the level of the lesions in hemispheric coma.
- Midbrain coma: pupils are dilated. The parasympathetic innervation to the pupil travels from the Edinger-Westphal nucleus in the dorsal midbrain with CN III to the pupilloconstrictor muscle. Hence, a lesion here leads to a dilated, sluggishly reactive pupil on the same side of the lesion.
- Pontine coma: pupils are pinpoints. The sympathetic fibers travel down from the hypothalamus and medially in the RAS; their lesioning leaves the midbrain's pupilloconstrictor unopposed.
- Medullary coma: pupils may be spared from any change. By this level the descending oculosympathetic tract has moved laterally to

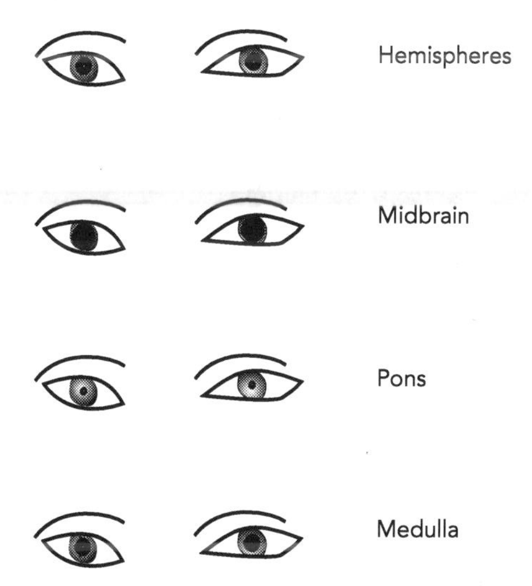

Figure 4.5 Pupil sizes in coma associated with lesions at specific levels.

synapse on the intermediolateral horn cells of the thoracolumbar spinal cord. Lesions of the medulla causing coma, affecting the midline reticular activating system, may spare the laterally placed descending oculosympathetic tracks, and thus the pupils are not necessarily affected. Alternatively, if a patient has dilated pupils during the herniation process stemming from midbrain involvement and continues to deteriorate with progressive brainstem impairment, the pupils tend to remain large.

The sympathetic fibers to the eye leave the upper thoracic segments of spinal cord and synapse in the superior cervical ganglion. From here they travel along the internal carotid artery, into the cavernous sinus, and then join the ophthalmic division of the trigeminal nerve (CN V). They enter the eye through the superior orbital fissure with the long ciliary nerves and innerve the iris dilator muscle (cf. Figure 4.19).

- Caveat: drugs can do anything. There are pupillodilators (anticholinergics, cocaine, and stimulants) and pupilloconstrictors (barbiturates, benzodiazepines, and sedative hypnotics).

■ Extraocular movements

There are two ways to test extraocular movements in the comatose patient: doll's eyes and cold calorics.

- Doll's eyes are the oculocephalic reflex (i.e., move the head and watch the eyes). They should float from side to side as long as the patient is comatose and unable to fix gaze. If they do not float fully, the calorics will provide a stronger stimulus to achieve eye movement. If there is concern about neck trauma and cervical spine radiographs have not been done to rule out a spine fracture, defer on doll's eyes. Remember, the normal doll's eyes float in the socket like the fancy dolls in the store, not the dolls where the eyes are glued, taped, or drawn.
- The calorics represent the oculovestibular, or vestibulo-ocular reflex (i.e., stimulate the vestibular system and watch the eyes). Here, ice cold water is placed in the ears. This discussion focuses on horizontal eye movements with the patient's head at a slight 30° elevation to align the horizontal semicircular canals.

When the cold water is applied to the tympanic membrane, there is freezing out, or inhibition, of the CN VIII input to the contralateral paramedian pontine reticular formation (PPRF), the horizontal gaze center adjacent to the CN VI nucleus. Hence, the eyes lose their influence to look contralaterally from that ear, and the other PPRF (ipsilateral to the injected ear) dominates, causing gaze to the injected side. In other words, *the eyes should look toward the ice*. If they do, the integrity of the entire brainstem, from the upper medulla to the midbrain, has been checked and is intact. If the eyes do anything else, one must deduce where the deficit lies. Calorics are a superb bedside technique to test the integrity of the brainstem in a comatose patient.

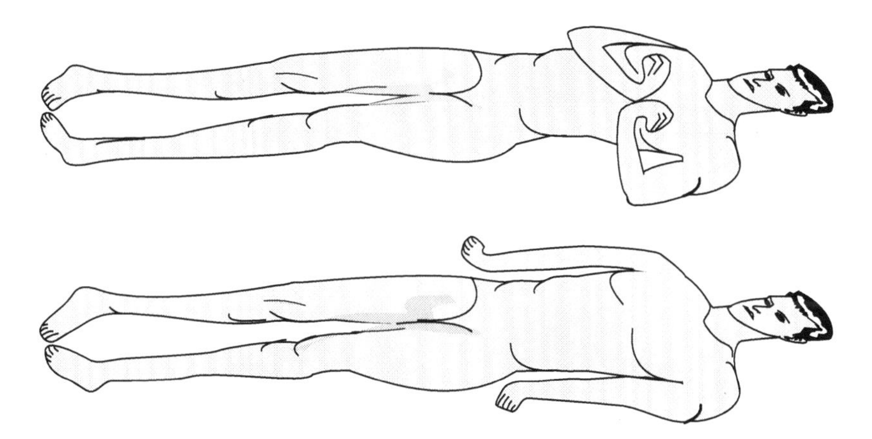

Figure 4.6 Decorticate (top panel, upper extremities triple flexed, lower extremities extended) versus decerebrate posturing (bottom panel, upper and lower extremities are both extended).

Note: There is no nystagmus in the comatose patient because nystagmus represents a compensatory response (as if to say, "Hey, get your eyes back on the road.") that is not available to the comatose patient.

- Motor

  Assess for asymmetries and posturing. Observe for spontaneous movement and motor responses to noxious stimulation.

  - Decorticate posturing—triple flexion of contralateral upper extremity involving the elbow, wrist, and metacarpophalangeal (MP) joints, along with pronation; the lower extremity extends. The lesion is from the cortex to the midbrain at about the level of the red nucleus.
  - Decerebrate posturing—extension, adduction, and internal rotation of the contralateral upper and lower extremities, involving all four extremities if bilateral. This implies dysfunction from the midbrain level down to the pontomedullary junction (Figure 4.6).
  - Flaccid paralysis—typical motor response associated with lesions below pontomedullary junction.

- Putting it all together:

  If the examination findings add up (i.e., mental status = comatose; respirations = apneustic; pupils = small; extraocular movements = impaired; and motor = decerebrate posturing), then one has localized the lesion(s) to a level (i.e., pons).

  If the examination findings are not so consistent, the localization is most likely multifocal, in which case the etiology is most often metabolic as opposed to structural.

  If the examination findings are deteriorating over time—from clouding of consciousness to stupor to coma; from eupneic respirations to hyperventilating; increasingly sluggish reactive and enlarging pupil; development of decorticate or decerebrate posturing—then one needs to be concerned with progressive deterioration and, hence, cerebral herniation.

B. BRAIN DEATH

1. Overview

There was a time when the doctor felt for a pulse or put his ear to the mouth to check for heart beat and respirations, respectively. If either was absent, the patient was declared dead.

Current technologies and the need to keep bodies alive for future organ use necessitate new definitions of death.

An individual with irreversible cessation of all function of the entire brain, including the brainstem, is dead. Setting up criteria to assess life or death of someone's brain is difficult. The Harvard Criteria (1968) established one of the first standard set of criteria for the diagnosis of brain death in adults.

2. Harvard Criteria

- *Unreceptive and unresponsive*
- *No movements or breathing*
- *No reflexes*
- *Flat electroencephalogram (EEG)*

In order to declare brain death, the tests noted should be repeated after 24 hours to confirm persistence of these findings. The presence of any central nervous system (CNS) depressant medications or hypothermia must be excluded because these are reversible yet can lead to these same clinical observations.

3. Collaborative Studies

Since the publishing of the Harvard Criteria, other studies and criteria have generally omitted a laboratory test such as an EEG or cerebral blood flow study (although these can be used as confirmatory tests when clinically indicated). Most individual hospitals have their own policies on what criteria are necessary to determine brain death, and these vary among adults, children, and neonates (with criteria not established for prematures).

Prerequisites

All appropriate diagnostic and therapeutic procedures have been performed; and neither hypotension nor hypothermia, nor severe acid/base, electrolyte, nor endocrine abnormality are present at the time of the examination.

Examination criteria

Must be present for 30 minutes at least 6 hours after the onset of coma:

- Coma
- Dilated, unreactive pupils
- Apneic during apnea test
- Absent cephalic reflexes

Definitions

- Coma: absence of a localizing response to nociceptive stimulation
- Apnea: absence of spontaneous respiration while being administered 100% oxygen during which the pCO_2 climbs to approximately 60 mmHg or at least 20 points from baseline
- Absent cephalic reflexes—pupillary, corneal, oculocephalic (doll's eyes), oculovestibular (calorics), or others: oculoauditory, ciliospinal, snout, coughing, pharyngeal, swallowing
- If an EEG is used, electrocerebral inactivity requires the technically accurate demonstration of absence of electrocerebral potentials of 2 or more microvolts

C. SEIZURES AND EPILEPSY

The idea that electrical activity might be generated within the human body was first seriously entertained in the early 1800s. Richard Caton documented the generation of electrical currents by the brain in 1875.

Where does this electrical activity come from? It comes mainly from excitatory postsynaptic potentials (EPSPs) and inhibitory postsynaptic potentials (IPSPs) of pyramidal cells that create local shifts in field potentials over the surface of the cerebral cortex, thus creating *brain waves* (Figure 4.7).

Brain waves are routinely recorded from an array of electrodes placed on the scalp—and sometimes invasively directly over the brain or on depth electrodes inserted into the brain parenchyma—producing the EEG. A seizure, coined from a Latin term meaning to take over (as when Sparta militarily seized Troy in the Peloponnesian wars), in modern medical parlance means that the brain has been taken over by an electrical event or storm.

1. Definitions and Concepts

Seizure

A paroxysmal, uncontrollable discharge of CNS neurons causing clinical signs and symptoms that interfere with normal function.

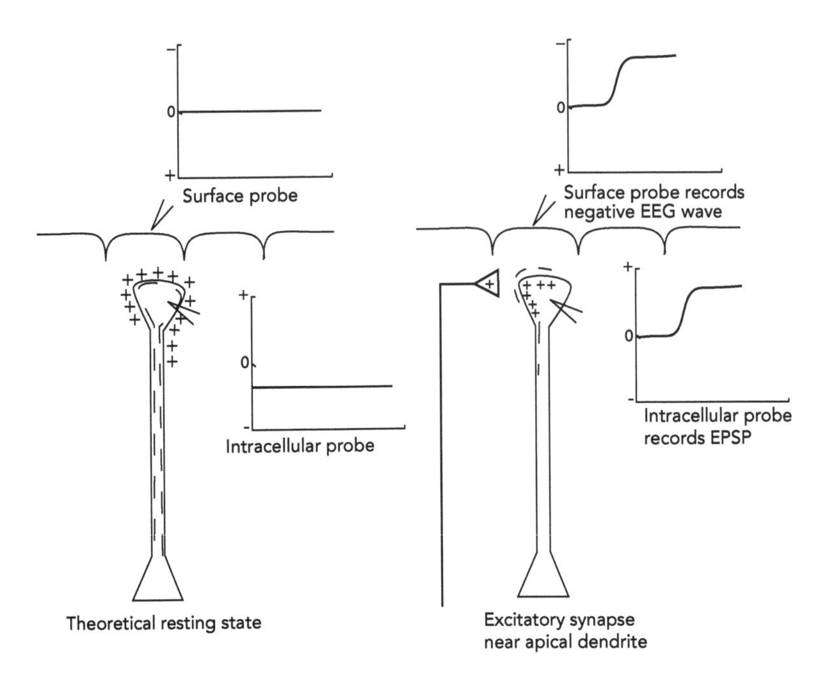

Figure 4.7 Electrophysiology of EPSPs, produced by depolarization of an apical dendrite. When a large population of neurons has EPSPs, they may summate into an epileptic discharge, or spike.

Epilepsy

Derived from a Greek term meaning recurrent events, denotes a neurological disorder characterized by spontaneous, recurrent seizures.

Epileptiform

A set of EEG patterns applied to waves or complexes distinguishable from the background activity, including spike and sharp waves, alone or accompanied by slow waves, occurring as isolated or repetitive discharges. Interictal epileptiform patterns are seen on EEGs between seizures, and EEG changes during actual seizure events are instead known as ictal patterns.

Pathophysiology

Overall, seizures are divided into focal (or partial) and generalized seizures.

- Focal onset seizures (previously also called "partial" although with new terminology discouraging use of the term *partial*, to avoid confusing a seizure as being something that can be partial versus complete)—presence of a seizure focus: Here there is a focus or zone of neurons with abnormal intrinsic properties that cause them to undergo excessive electrical discharges. This activity may continue to spread, thus causing a secondarily generalized seizure.

There may be an aura, or warning, prior to a focal seizure. Aura is taken from the Greek word meaning breeze (i.e., the breeze before the storm). This represents the first phase of the seizure. In classical migraine headaches, the term is also used to signify the earliest phase of the migraine that may be represented by an aura of vision loss or focal numbness or weakness.

- Primary generalized seizures—corticoreticular theory (Figure 4.8): Previously conceptualized as the centrencephalic theory, positing that the thalamus is the central pacemaker to generate primary generalized seizures, the corticoreticular theory invokes the important role of two oscillating centers, the cerebral cortex and the subcortical reticular activating system and thalamus. These cortical and subcortical structures become synchronized, causing generalized epileptiform activity on EEGs. Thus, normal cerebral function is interrupted, which may cause abrupt loss of consciousness (e.g., petit mal or absence seizures), convulsions (generalized tonic–clonic seizures), or other generalized seizures (e.g., myoclonic, tonic, atonic).

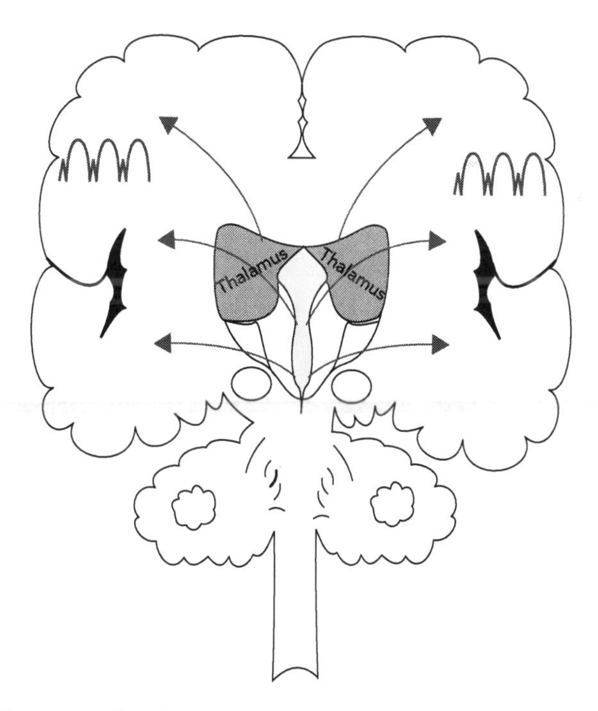

Figure 4.8 Generalized seizures are thought to reflect interaction between the central thalamic pacemaker, producing a generalized spike-wave as shown here, and the cerebral cortex.

2. Differential Diagnosis of Seizures

- *Febrile seizures* (ages 1 month–5 years)

Toxic/metabolic

- Alcohol or barbiturate withdrawal
- Drug toxicity (e.g., lidocaine, aminophylline, or penicillin overdose)
- Hypocalcemia, hypoglycemia, hypomagnesemia, or hyponatremia
- Organ system dysfunction: Hashimoto's thyroiditis, uremia, or hepatic encephalopathy

Infections

- Meningitis
- Encephalitis
- Subdural empyema
- Brain abscess

Neoplastic

- Primary CNS tumors (e.g., meningiomas, or gliomas)
- Cerebral metastases
- Carcinomatous meningitis
- Paraneoplastic syndromes (e.g., limbic encephalitis)

Congenital

- Structural brain malformations (e.g., porencephaly, or migrational brain anomalies)
- Perinatal encephalopathy

Degenerative

- Poliodystrophies (gray matter diseases of infancy and childhood, e.g., Tay Sachs disease, neuronal ceroid lipofuscinosis) are more likely to have seizures early in their course than primarily white matter diseases, known as leukodystrophies.
- Alzheimer disease may include seizures (5%–10%).
- Multiple sclerosis (although a disease of white matter, lesions at the gray/white junction may cause neuronal dysfunction [less than 10%]).

Trauma

- Following closed-head injury: acute (first 24 hours), early (1 day–7 days), late
- Additional risk factors: parenchymal brain contusion, hematoma (epidural, subdural), depressed skull fracture

Vascular/collagen vascular

- Arteriovascular malformations
- Stroke (typically embolic when seizure occurs at onset)
- Postinfarction (6 months–2 years following event)
- Autoimmune diseases (e.g., lupus, polyarteritis nodosa, primary cerebral vasculitis)

3. Epilepsy

Epilepsy is a syndrome of recurring seizures that can be caused by any of the disorders discussed in the preceding section. All individuals have a *seizure threshold* that can be aggravated by sleep deprivation, fatigue, hypoglycemia, head trauma, fever, drugs, and genetics. Traditionally, epilepsy syndromes have been classified as idiopathic (of presumably genetic cause without other stigmata of brain dysfunction), cryptogenic (of hidden but suspected cause in the presence of brain dysfunction), and symptomatic (caused by an underlying brain disorder). This classification system is being revamped because of blurred distinctions among these entities—for example, gene mutations causing any of a variety of conditions that previously may have been considered idiopathic, cryptogenic, or symptomatic disorders that in some cases involve the same gene!

Clinical classification of epileptic seizures

- Focal seizures:
  - No impairment of consciousness (formerly called simple partial seizures)
    - Focal motor
    - Focal sensory
    - Autonomic
    - Psychic
  - Associated impairment of consciousness (formerly called complex partial seizures, and termed "focal dyscognitive" seizures)
- Generalized seizures:
  - Absence (synonymous with petit mal)
  - Tonic–clonic (synonymous with grand mal or major motor seizure)
  - Clonic
  - Tonic
  - Myoclonic (formerly called minor motor seizure)
  - Atonic
- Unclassifiable:
  - Neonatal seizures
  - Infantile spasms

Conditions mimicking epilepsy

- Breath-holding attacks (children ages 6 months–6 years, cyanotic type after fit of crying versus pallid infantile type after fright or head bump); benign and outgrown
- Night terrors (onset 2 years–10 years); partial arousal from deep sleep
- Syncope (fainting-related vasovagal fit, orthostasis, cardiac causes)
- Psychogenic (conversion disorder; do not expect to see loss of consciousness, tongue biting, incontinence, injury from fall, postictal drowsiness; eyes are usually open in an epileptic seizure but may be open or closed in a psychogenic seizure)
- Cataplexy (loss of motor tone which may lead to a fall, following an emotional surge or suprise, without a loss of consciousness)

Localization of seizures: typical behavioral features of seizures from specific areas

- Temporal lobe:
  - Medial hippocampal-amygdalar origin: strange sensation, rising epigastric discomfort, nausea, fear, panic, belching, pallor, facial fullness or flushing, respiratory arrest, pupillary dilatation
  - Lateral neocortical temporal origin: auditory or visual hallucinations, illusions, dreamy states, vertigo, aphasia if dominant hemisphere
  - May begin with motor arrest, followed by oroalimentary automatisms and autonomic phenomena
  - Typical duration of more than 1 minute, followed by postictal confusion
- Frontal lobe:
  - Primary motor cortex: unilateral clonic activity, Jacksonian (details in Chapter 2) march
  - Supplementary motor cortex: posturing (e.g., fencing), focal tonic, vocalization or speech arrest
  - Cingulate cortex: changes in mood and affect, vegetative signs, elaborate gestural automatisms
  - Orbitofrontal cortex: olfactory hallucinations and illusions, gestural automatisms, autonomic signs
  - Dorsolateral cortex: tonic or clonic signs, versive eye and head movements
  - Typically brief, often nocturnal, urinary incontinence, minimal postictal confusion
- Parietal lobe:
  - Somatosensory signs and symptoms, intra-abdominal sensation of sinking, choking, nausea, numbness, rarely pain, may have rotary or postural movements
  - Dominant parietal lobe: language disturbances

- Nondominant parietal lobe: asomatognosia (loss of awareness of part or half of body), disorientation, vertigo

- Occipital lobe:
  - Visual symptoms: negative (scotoma, hemianopia, amaurosis) or positive (sparks or flashes, illusions, hallucinations)
  - Tonic or clonic activity of eyes and head, or oculoclonic or oculogyric deviation of the eyes
  - Headache

- Multilobar:
  - Perirolandic: motor and/or sensory especially in face, tongue, and hand
    - If lower perirolandic: speech arrest, vocalization, dysphasia, swallowing, tongue sensations, stiffness, coldness
    - If pericentral lobule: contralateral lower extremity sensory symptoms, lateralized genital sensations, tonic movements of either foot
  - Opercular (perisylvian, insular): mastication/chewing, salivation, swallowing, laryngeal symptoms, epigastric sensations, fear, vegetative phenomena, clonic facial movements, numbness in hands, bilateral upper extremity movements
  - Temporal-parietal-occipital junction: visual illusions (include micropsia, macropsia, teleopsia, distortion of objects) and hallucinations (complex, may see one's own image or autoscopy), other hallucinations (auditory, olfactory, gustatory, autonomic), vertigo
  - Hypothalamic: gelastic (eerie giggling or laughter)

D. MOVEMENT

1. Conceptualization

Movement results from an intricate system of excitatory and inhibitory signals impacting on a group of muscles at a particular point in time. The origination and transmission of a signal from the CNS to muscles must occur to generate movement. What is the neural basis for this?

Initially there may be a thought, at least to generate voluntary movement. Conceptualization of an idea takes place in an undetermined cerebral locale, probably with bilateral representation, and likely at least involves the limbic system. Then, impulses arrive at the primary motor cortex, Brodmann (details in Chapter 2) area 4 (Figure 2.2) appropriate for that particular movement (i.e., right lower motor strip for left-hand movement).

The cerebral cortex has six layers, with layer 1 being the most superficial and layer 6 the deepest (Figure 4.9):

1. Molecular
2. External granular
3. External pyramidal
4. Internal granular
5. Internal pyramidal
6. Multiform

The pyramidal cells, which begin the pyramidal or corticospinal tracts, are located in layer 3 and layer 5. The motor cortex is particularly thick in these layers, especially layer 5. These neurons are activated and, furthermore, receive information from the parietal, occipital, and temporal lobes, the cerebellum, and the basal ganglia. Input from the parietal lobes provides necessary information about the location of the limb, not only in space but with respect to the rest of the body. Temporal connections allow for audio feedback, and occipitofrontal projections coordinate visual-motor integration. Modulation of motor output by the cerebellum and basal ganglia via the thalamus ensures smooth execution of each movement.

Immediately anterior to the primary motor strip is Brodmann area 6, an accessory motor area where preprogrammed movement sequences are stored. If one decides to walk up a flight of stairs, this area's *stepping sequence* is initiated in addition to the pyramidal cells in the primary motor strip. There are many interneurons and glial elements that modify the output of the pyramidal tracts; the corticospinal tract consists of more than 1 million fibers, of which only 30,000 to 40,000 represent axons of pyramidal cells.

The corticospinal tracts pass from the cortex through the subcortical white matter as the centrum semiovale, and then the genu and posterior limb

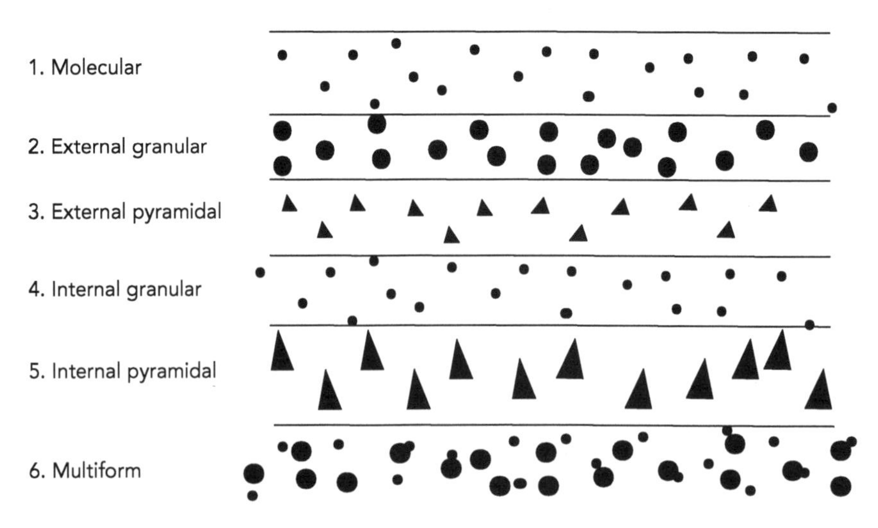

Figure 4.9 Six layers of the cerebral cortex.

of the internal capsule and through the brainstem as the ventral peduncles of the midbrain, basis pontis of the pons, and medullary pyramids. Throughout the brainstem, frontobulbar fibers traveling with the corticospinal tracts branch off at their appropriate levels to synapse on pontine relay nuclei and the cranial nerve nuclei. At the cervicomedullary junction there is decussation of 75% to 90% of the fibers, forming the lateral corticospinal tracts of the spinal cord. The remaining uncrossed fibers, innervating the truncal musculature, form the anterior corticospinal tracts and a small uncrossed portion of the lateral corticospinal tract.

There is medial to lateral organization within the corticospinal tracts, with leg fibers remaining lateral, trunk fibers intermediate, and arm fibers most medial. At the appropriate spinal level, axons leave the corticospinal tract and enter the anterior horns synapsing on both interneurons and, ultimately, the anterior horn cells of the ventral horn of the spinal cord gray matter. These cells also receive input from sensory receptors in the periphery, muscle spindles, spinal reflexes, and other descending extrapyramidal tracts (i.e., rubrospinal, reticulospinal, and vestibulospinal tracts) (Figure 4.10).

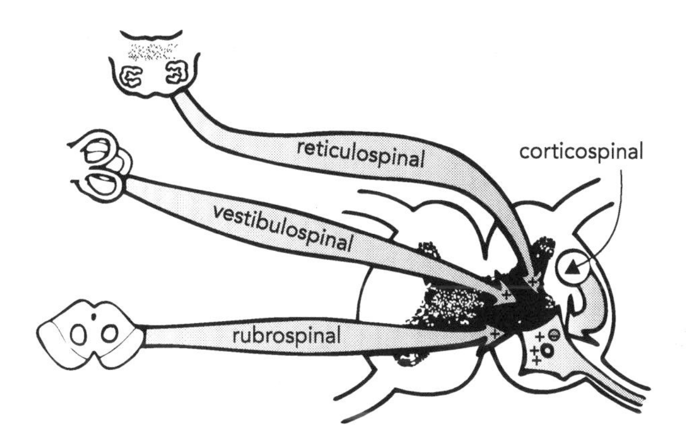

Figure 4.10 LMN inputs.

The anterior horn cells integrate this information and discharge a signal down their axons, which exit as the anterior spinal roots. In the cervical and lumbosacral regions there is intermixing of these root fibers forming the brachial and lumbosacral plexuses, from which emerge the peripheral nerves to the arms and legs.

Motor axons have specialized terminals where packets, or vesicles, of acetylcholine are stored. With depolarization of the motor nerve terminal in the presence of calcium, acetylcholine is released into the neuromuscular junction and diffuses across the synaptic cleft to react with specialized acetylcholine receptors on the muscle end plate. With adequate depolarization of the muscle end plate, the contractile sequence of the muscle fibers is initiated. At the same time that any one muscle is being activated, a similar sequence of events ensures contraction of agonist and inhibition of antagonistic muscles at synergistic joints.

2. Disorders of Movement: Upper Versus Lower Motor Neuron Syndromes

Overview

Neurons from the cerebral cortex all the way to presynaptic neurons innervating the anterior horn cells are called upper motor neurons, or sometimes premotor neurons, and lesions of these are associated clinically with upper motor neuron syndromes. The anterior horn cell that projects onto muscle fibers, all of which are known as a motor unit, is known as the lower motor neuron, or sometimes just as motor neuron. Lesions of this motor unit produce clinically lower motor neuron syndromes. Following are the clinical hallmarks of upper motor (or premotor) versus lower motor (or motor) neuron syndromes (see image of upper versus lower motor neuron signs at the top of page 65).

Upper motor neuron syndromes

- Hypertonicity (clasp-knife spasticity for pyramidal tract lesions; cogwheel rigidity for extrapyramidal lesions; may be initially flaccid in a large lesion)
- Hyperreflexia (applies to the deep tendon reflexes, which may be absent initially for a large lesion; if superficial reflexes are involved, they are lost in upper or lower motor neuron lesions—examples: blink, gag, periumbilical, cremasteric, anal wink)
- Extensor plantar response
- Clonus (repeated contraction and relaxation of the muscle triggered by a single stretch of the muscle tendon reflex, designated as 4+)

Lower motor neuron syndromes

- Weakness (more severe than in upper motor neuron lesions)
- Flaccid tone
- Muscle atrophy
- Hyporeflexia
- Fasciculations (flickering of muscle, as experienced commonly in the nondominant upper eyelid with fatigue, but pathologic when involving large muscle groups and associated with weakness)

Features of syndromes based on localization of lesion

- Cortical lesion:
  - Left hemisphere typically associated with aphasia (virtually all right-handers and close to 80% of left-handers are L hemisphere dominant for language)
  - Homonymous visual field cuts (see Figure 2.23)
  - Cortical pattern of sensory loss—parietal lobe signs
  - Agnosia (e.g., left hemineglect in right parietal lesions)
  - Apraxia—impaired execution of complex motor tasks
  - Dissociation of weakness (e.g., face and arm weaker than leg [F, A, greater than L] in MCA [middle cerebral artery] stroke versus leg

weaker than face and arm [L greater than F, A] in ACA [anterior cerebral artery] stroke (see Figure 2.5)

- Internal capsule:

  May be small discrete lacunae, or islands of involvement, resulting in restricted deficits (e.g., pure motor or pure sensory). Yet face, arm, and leg may be equally affected due to the close proximity of the pyramidal tract fibers (i.e., F = A = L). The classic lacunar stroke syndromes are:
  - Pure hemisensory loss
  - Pure hemiplegia
  - Hemiparesis with ipsilateral cerebellar signs (ataxic hemiparesis)
  - Dysarthria–clumsy hand

- Brainstem:

  Although any combination of symptoms may be seen with propagation of a clot in the vertebrobasilar system, several classical brainstem vascular syndromes have been described. They may occasionally be mimicked by tumors or encephalitis, but rarely in their pure form. Following (Figures 4.11–4.15; Tables 4.1–4.5) are some of the classic brainstem stroke syndromes, along with their clinical features, structures involved, and eponyms.

Table 4.1 Weber Syndrome (Ventral Midbrain)*

Signs and symptoms†	Structures involved
Ipsilateral CN III palsy	CN III fibers
Contralateral hemiplegia	Corticospinal tract (cerebral peduncle)

*First described in 1863.

†See Figure 4.11.

Abbreviation: CN, cranial nerve

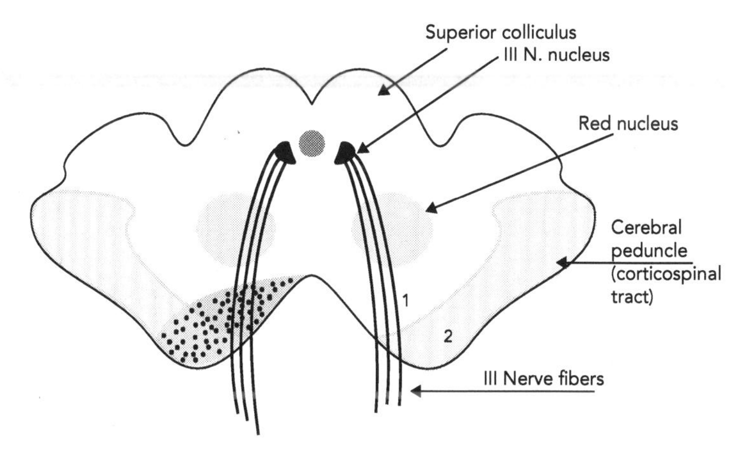

Figure 4.11 Weber syndrome (1863) of the ventral midbrain.

Table 4.2 Benedikt Syndrome (Paramedian Midbrain)*

Signs and symptoms†	Structures involved
Ipsilateral CN III palsy	CN III fibers
Contralateral hemiplegia	Corticospinal tract (cerebral peduncle)
Contralateral tremor	Cerebellothalamic fibers passing through the red nucleus

*First described in 1872.
†See Figure 4.12.
Abbreviation: CN, cranial nerve.

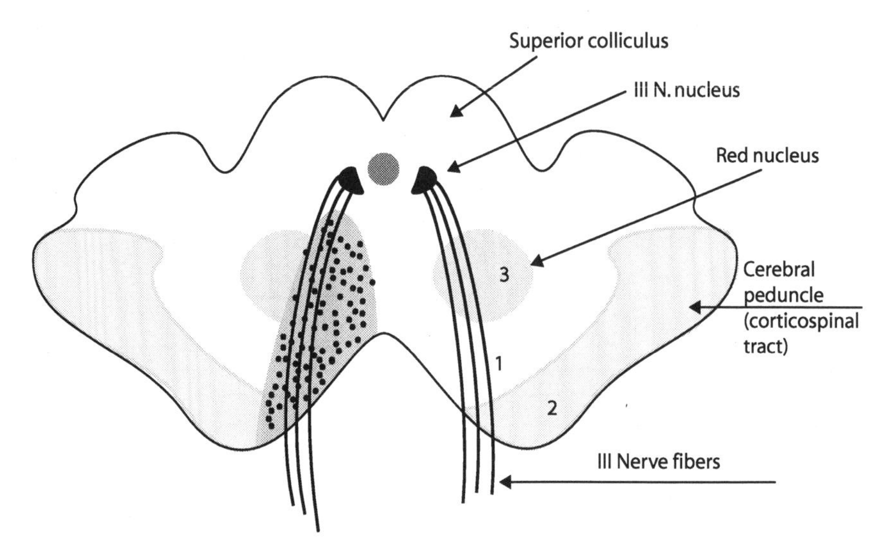

Figure 4.12 Benedikt syndrome (1872) of the paramedian midbrain.

Table 4.3 Millard-Gubler Syndrome (Median/Paramedian Pons)*

Signs and symptoms†	Structures involved
Ipsilateral facial palsy (peripheral type)	Facial nerve (CN VII)
Ipsilateral ocular abduction loss	Abducens nerve (CN VI)
Contralateral hemiparesis (below face)	Corticospinal tract (basis pontis)

*First described in 1858.
†See Figure 4.13.
Abbreviation: CN, cranial nerve.

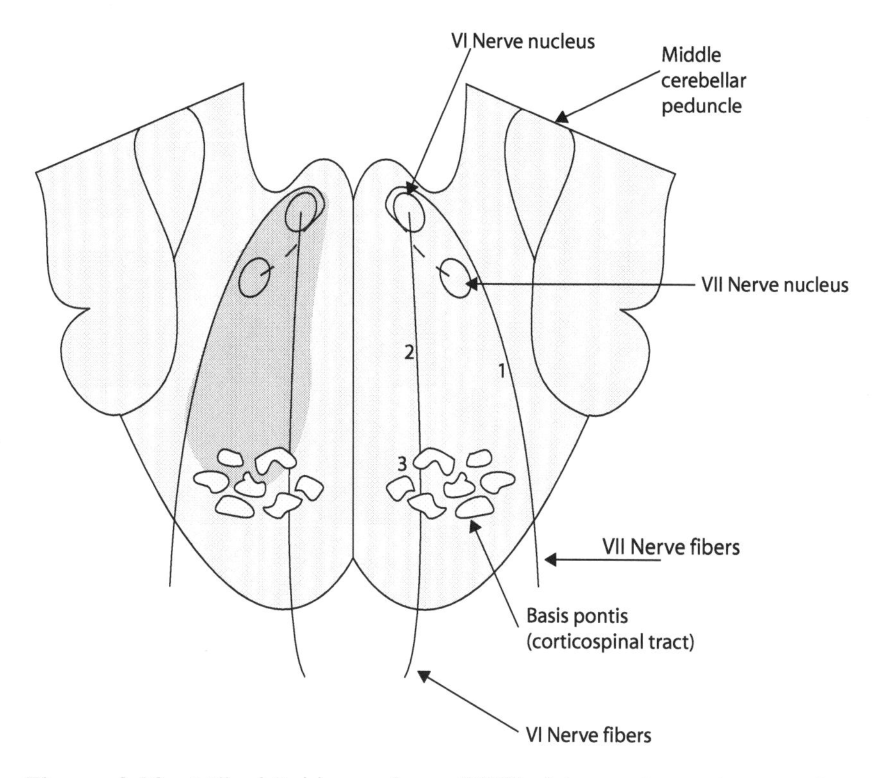

Figure 4.13 Millard-Gubler syndrome (1858) of the median and paramedian pons.

Table 4.4 Wallenberg Syndrome (Lateral Medullary Plate Syndrome, Occlusion of Vertebral Artery Affecting the Distribution of the Posterior Inferior Cerebellar Artery [PICA])*

Signs and symptoms†	Structures involved
Ipsilateral facial numbness	CN V nucleus and tract
Ipsilateral ataxia	Inferior cerebellar peduncle
Nausea, vomiting, vertigo	Vestibular nuclei
Ipsilateral Horner syndrome	Descending oculosympathetic tract
Dysphagia, hoarseness	Nucleus ambiguous (affects CNs IX and X)
Palatal myoclonus	Central tegmental tract, from solitary nerve
Contralateral body loss of pain, temperature	Lateral spinothalamic tract

*First described in 1895.

†See Figure 4.14.

Abbreviation: CN, cranial nerve.

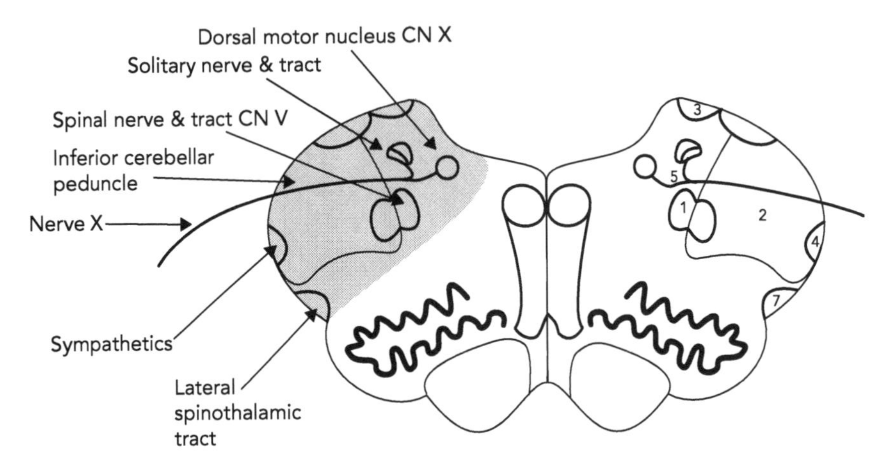

Figure 4.14 Wallenberg syndrome of the lateral medulla.

Table 4.5 Dejerine Medial Medullary Syndrome (Occlusion of Anterior Spinal Artery)*

Signs and symptoms†	Structures involved
Contralateral hemiplegia	Corticospinal tracts
Contralateral hemisensory (position, vibration sense)	Medial lemniscus
Ipsilateral tongue weakness	Hypoglossal nerve

*First described in 1914.

†See Figure 4.15.

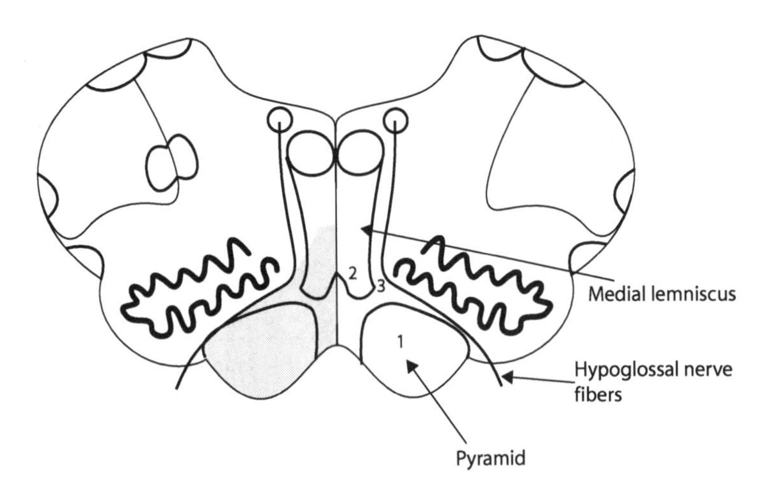

Figure 4.15 Dejerine syndrome of the medial medulla.

- Spinal cord corticospinal tracts:
  - Normal examination above the level of the lesion
  - Face always spared
  - Typical characteristics of upper motor neuron injury below the level of the lesion

Note: At the level of the lesion, if the anterior horn cells as well as descending long tracts are involved, there may be corresponding lower motor neuron segmental atrophy and hyporeflexia at the specific level involved, in addition to upper motor neuron findings below the level of the lesion. For example, in the case of C7, C8 cervical spondylosis causing a cartilaginous spur to affect the lower cervical spinal cord, there may be:

  - Atrophy and weakness of the intrinsic muscles of the hand, particularly those with ulnar innervation (C8)
  - Symptoms corresponding to lower motor neuron injury (C7, C8)
  - Decreased triceps reflex
  - Increased tone and reflexes in the *lower* extremities
  - Weakness in lower extremities

Bulbar and pseudobulbar palsy

The bulb is the classic term for the brainstem. Certain disease processes have a propensity to involve this region producing recognizable signs, thus warranting its separation as a distinct clinical syndrome.

- Bulbar palsy:

  The brainstem is analogous to the spinal cord in a simplistic sense in that it houses the lower motor neurons for facial movement in the same way the spinal cord contains similar cells for arm, leg, and trunk movements.

  Disease processes such as poliomyelitis, amyotrophic lateral sclerosis (ALS), and proximal motor nerve roots (Guillain-Barré syndrome) that selectively involve anterior horn cells may produce bulbar palsy (in addition to spinal cord involvement).

  Clinically, bulbar palsy manifests with decreased strength, tone, and bulk in muscles innervated by CN nuclei. There is impairment in facial movement, speech, and swallowing. The jaw jerk and gag reflexes are decreased.

- Pseudobulbar palsy:

  In pseudobulbar palsy, the lesion affects corticobulbar tracks, linking the cerebral cortex to the CN nuclei. This produces an upper motor neuron pattern of bulbar dysfunction, and results in exaggerated smiling and crying facial expressions (also known as emotional incontinence) as well as increased jaw jerk and gag reflexes. There is often accompanying spasticity of speech due to inability to coordinate respiratory and vocal cord functions. The patient has difficulty modulating the tone of voice and tends to shout in short bursts irregularly interrupted by respiration. An example of a process causing pseudobulbar palsy is multiple small lacunar infarctions associated with long-standing hypertension. This is also seen in patients with cerebral palsy having long-standing diffuse motor dysfunction. Frontal lobe release signs may also be present.

Frontal lobe release signs

Classical neurologists have long noted that reflexes considered to be normal during the neonatal and infantile periods of development may return later in life under conditions of neurological disease. The frontal lobe release signs are so named because these patterned motor responses are suppressed when myelination of the frontal lobes occurs in the first 2 years of life; their reappearance later in life represents a disinhibition or release from control.

The snout, rooting, sucking, and grasp responses in neonates are protective and adaptive. Following are examples of frontal lobe release signs and methods to elicit them when evaluating patients for frontal lobe disease.

- Snout:

  Place finger over or just above the patient's lips and tap gently—patient responds by puckering up.

- Suck:

  Place tongue depressor in patient's mouth—patient sucks it (the suck reflex may be so strong in patients with pseudobulbar palsy that they cannot push food to the back of the palate to swallow, and instead chew one bolus of food ad infinitum).

- Grasp:

  Stroke palm of patient's hand as though you were going to shake hands while instructing the patient not to hold on—patient grasps hand.

- Palmomental reflex:

  Stroke palm of patient's hand with somewhat noxious stimulus (e.g., wooden end of swab)—ipsilateral contraction of patient's mentalis muscle (chin).

Gait disorders

Gait is an excellent screen of a patient's motor functioning and should be assessed as a routine part of the neurological examination. Typically the patient should be asked to demonstrate routine gait as well as heel, toe, and tandem (heel to toe) gait. The description of gait caused by lesions at each level of the neuraxis is given in the sections following, starting in a reverse rostrocaudal direction (i.e., from the most peripheral levels of the motor system).

- Muscle disease: *myopathy—waddling gait:*

  Muscle disease tends to produce more proximal than distal muscle group weakness. The classic example here is the boy with Duchenne muscular dystrophy who has hypertrophic calves, lordotic posture, and a waddling gait.

- Neuromuscular junction disease—*fatigable gait:*

  The cardinal junction disease is myasthenia gravis. Although these patients do not generally present with a primary complaint of gait disturbance, the hallmark of these conditions is fatigue, and one would characterize their motor difficulties—especially diplopia, ptosis, and overall weakness—as having a prominent component of fatigue, as well as some recovery with rest.

- Peripheral nerve disease: *neuropathy—steppage gait:*

  Peripheral neuropathy typically causes more distal than proximal muscle group weakness, in contrast to myopathies. In peripheral neuropathy, one would often see peroneal nerve impairment leading to drop foot. Hence, a patient will have a *slap* or *steppage* gait where the toe falls before the heel, similar to the hoof of a horse.

  Another aspect of peripheral neuropathy may be proprioceptive loss, where patients have difficulty identifying the location of a particular foot in space. This can be further tested with the Romberg examination: A patient stands with eyes closed, and falling is caused by proprioceptive loss once vision is reduced. This may be called *sensory ataxia* to denote gait difficulty caused by loss of position sense, as opposed to true ataxia associated with dysfunction of the cerebellum or cerebellar outflow tracks (see cerebellar disease section following).

- Root disease: *radiculopathy—antalgic gait:*

  Root disease, when caused by a herniated disc or mass lesion affecting the nerve root(s) such as metastases, is associated with pain in the distribution of the nerve root's pattern of innervation. This is known as an antalgic gait, referring to the presence of pain.

- Spinal cord disease: *myelopathy—scissoring gait:*

  Here we are transitioning from the lower motor neuron to the upper motor neuron lesions, and thus lesioned white matter descending tracks lead to prominent spasticity, causing the legs to be so stiff they may cross like scissors as the patient ambulates. Naturally, the associated neurological findings can vary when the cord syndrome, known as a myelopathy, more prominently affects the descending corticospinal motor tracks versus the anterior horn cells versus the dorsal horns or other structures.

- Basal ganglia disease: hyperkinetic disorders—*dancing gait:*

  Basal ganglia diseases can be viewed in a number of different ways, from descriptive terminology (i.e., the classical movement disorders: tic, myoclonus, chorea, athetosis, ballismus, and stereotypy) to an emphasis on rate of movement because the basal ganglia have significant control over our speed. The disorders may be differentiated as hyperkinetic (i.e., Huntington chorea or Sydenham chorea) or hypokinetic (i.e., Parkinson disease). Sydenham chorea, a poststreptococcal complication that is pathognomonic of acute rheumatic fever, presents with a form of proximal chorea often known as St. Vitus's dance—based on early descriptions during the Middle Ages of patients afflicted with this disease.

- Hypokinetic disorders—*festinate gait:*

  In the case of hypokinetic disorders such as Parkinson disease, the cardinal manifestations are resting tremor, cogwheel rigidity, brady kinesia, and gait instability. There is a stooped posture, the gait appears shuffling, and the patient cannot actually come to a stop easily, described as a festinating or festinate gait.

- Cerebellar disease—*ataxia:*

  The cerebellum is the great modulator of the nervous system. It reduces many of the perturbations. Cerebellar disease is assessed on examination by looking for the presence of nystagmus, intention tremor, impaired rapid alternating or sequential movements (known as dysdiadochokinesia), heel-knee-shin tremor, and gait ataxia. Here is where the neurologist means ataxia (i.e., pertaining to the cerebellum and its pathways). A cerebellar gait is a wide-based gait. Normally the knees, or at least pant legs, should nearly brush against each other during routine gait. Tandem gait—where the patient walks in a straight line, touching the toe to the heel—is typically relied on to test for cerebellar ataxia. The policeman uses the same method when assessing for effects of alcohol, which preferentially affects the vermis of the cerebellar midline and provides motor control to the legs.

- Hemispheric disease—*circumductive gait:*

  The presence of a hemispheric lesion affecting the corticospinal track affects the extremities in a certain pattern—more upper extremity extensor weakness and hence a stiff and flexed upper extremity, and more lower extremity flexor weakness and hence a stiff, extended lower extremity. This leads to the circumductive gait, where a patient has difficulty even bending the knee while walking and has to swing it around, producing the appearance of circumduction.

- Frontal lobe disease: *apraxia—magnetic gait:*

  Apraxia is characterized by the inability to perform a complex motor task. An example would be the older patient with normal pressure hydrocephalus, which presents with the triad of dementia, urinary incontinence, and gait apraxia. Here, the patient's feet appear to be stuck to the floor. The patient may be able to lie in bed and exert normal group muscle strength; however, once placed on the ground, the feet act like magnets implanted on the floor, and hence the term magnetic gait.

- Psychiatric disease: *conversion disorder—astasia abasia:*

  At one time, gait was quantified on the basis of *station* and *base.* The term astasia abasia is often used to connote patients who have no stability or clear base to their gait, but who otherwise have no neurological deficit other than sometimes the la belle indifference associated with conversion disorders.

- *Multifactorial gait:*

  Clinically, gait dysfunction cannot always be localized to one level, and may result from multifactorial causes. This is especially true in older patients when there is a combination of some vision loss, hearing loss, and vertigo, peripheral neuropathy, and possibly dementia as well as nonneurologic factors. The gait difficulty that results from a variety of sources such as pain, orthopedic disease, rheumatologic conditions, or problems such as vascular claudication all must be considered within the context of what neurological deficits are present or absent to distinguish these from primary neurological disorders.

E. DIZZINESS AND VERTIGO

Vertigo is the illusory perception of oneself moving with respect to the environment or vice versa, analogous to the spinning feeling that lasts after a merry-go-round stops moving. The sensation of movement is not dependent on vision or associated nystagmus; blind patients and patients with complete oculomotor paralysis experience the spinning sensation comparable to that of normal subjects if the vestibular end organs are stimulated. Focal cortical lesions in the parietal lobe (usually nondominant) disturb spatial relations, and epileptic discharges may create the subjective illusion of movement. There is a cerebral cortical representation for vestibular sensation and it is here that labyrinthine, somatic proprioceptive, and visual signals are integrated to give a conscious awareness of body orientation, although these sensations usually only reach consciousness when they are disrupted and abnormal, thus creating dizziness and vertigo.

A review of the anatomy and physiology of the vestibular system is necessary for troubleshooting when a patient presents with vertigo. If you:

Tilt a newborn baby's head back, the eyes roll down to maintain gaze.
Shake your head from side to side as you read, the print stands still.
Drop a cat upside down, it lands upright.

These noted reflexes that we take for granted are representative of vestibular function. The sensory apparatus in the vestibule of the inner ear works actively to transduce the forces associated with head acceleration and gravity into a biological signal. Control centers of the brain use this signal to develop a subjective awareness of head position in relation to the environment (orientation) and to produce motor reflexes for equilibrium and locomotion.

1. Sense of Balance and Orientation

- Vestibular
- Visual
- Somatic (joint position etc.)

Vestibular sense is different from other senses (e.g., olfaction or vision) because it is only one component contributing to the system serving balance and orientation that also receives input from the visual system and somatic receptors. In addition, loss of one part of this system does not render it permanently nonfunctional.

There are two types of vestibular receptors:

- Otolith organs (utricles and saccules)—respond to linear acceleration (Definition: a change in the velocity of an object traveling in a straight line—includes action of gravity)
- Semicircular canals—respond to angular acceleration (Definition: change in rate of rotations)

The otoliths and semicircular canals work dynamically together serving the three major functions of vestibular sense.

Functional roles of vestibular reflexes

- To produce negative geotropic movement to compensate for changes in the direction of the force of gravity (so you don't collapse to the ground)
- To produce contractions of muscles for maintenance of equilibrium and importantly ocular stability during movement
- To help maintain posture and muscle tone (with direct excitatory input to alpha motor neurons via vestibulospinal tracts)

2. Vestibular Connections: Anatomy

These functions are made possible by a complex arrangement of interconnecting fibers among the vestibular nuclei, cerebellum, extraocular muscle nuclei, anterior horn cells, and cortical centers.

Vestibular nerves from the otoliths and semicircular canals enter the brainstem at the cerebellopontine angle and synapse in the vestibular nuclei that extend from the medulla to the pons. There is a resting baseline level of activity in each vestibular nerve. A small group of fibers bypass the vestibular nuclei, form the juxtarestiform body, and terminate directly in the flocculonodular lobe of the cerebellum—the vestibulocerebellum.

Secondary fibers project from the vestibular nuclei to:

- Cerebellum (mostly ipsilateral)
- Motor cranial nerve nuclei via MLF (medial longitudinal fasciculus) (crossed and uncrossed)
- All spinal levels (vestibulospinal tracts); strong excitatory influence on muscle tone, particularity extensor tone

Vestibular dysfunction is characterized by one or more of the following:

- Vertigo—the subjective sensation of movement
- Nystagmus
- Nausea and/or vomiting
- Unsteadiness in standing and walking
- Postural deviation—toward the side of the lesion in peripheral lesions
- Auditory symptoms—tinnitus, hearing loss, and sense of pressure or fullness in ear with lesions of vestibular end organ or nerve
- Brainstem neighborhood signs in the case of central causes

Magnitude of symptoms is determined by:

- Extent of the lesion
- Unilaterality versus bilaterality—patients who slowly lose bilateral vestibular function (i.e., with streptomycin toxicity) may not complain; however, when questioned they may report visual blurring (oscillopsia) with head movement, and instability when walking in the dark.
- Rapidity with which functional loss occurs:
  - Acute vestibular lesions are usually accompanied by the abrupt onset of symptoms that then decrease in intensity as compensation takes place.
  - Chronic vestibular disorders may occur in brief paroxysms or may have background dizziness with exacerbations.
  - Continuous dizziness without fluctuation for long periods of time is not typical of vestibular disorders.

3. Nystagmus

Nystagmus is a very helpful albeit confusing feature of vestibular system disease. Nystagmus is a rapid eye movement that may be classified by the direction of the movement. Figure 4.16 is a tic-tac-toe diagram depicting the eye movements depending on the direction of gaze. For example, in gaze evoked nystagmus, the movements are seen on the left when the patient gazes to the left, whereas in unidirectional nystagmus, the nystagmus is toward the left in all directions of gaze. There are only four types of normal physiologic nystagmus:

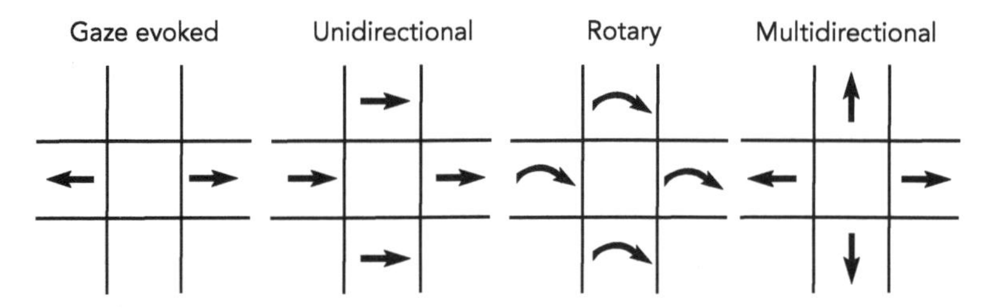

Figure 4.16 Nystagmus may be gaze evoked, occuring at the extremes of gaze, usually horizontal; unidirectional, beating in the same direction regardless of gaze; rotary with a torsional component; or multidirectional, beating in the direction of gaze. The direction of nystagmus is named for the rapid, corrective component.

- Caloric induced—with irrigation of the external auditory canal with warm or cool water
- Rotatory induced—by rotating a person in a chair
- Optokinetic—induced by a twirling drum of stripes or moving images (e.g., watching trees go by while riding in a moving car)
- End point—slight nystagmus seen at far lateral gaze

All other forms of nystagmus represent a pathological derangement of vestibular function (whether the dysfunction is based on peripheral or central localization) (Table 4.6).

Spontaneous vestibular nystagmus (peripheral)—characteristics:

- Unidirectional
- Usually has a rotatory component
- Inhibited by asking a patient to fixate on a target, except in the very acute stages
- Etiology: viral labyrinthitis, Ménière disease

Paroxysmal positional nystagmus (peripheral)—characteristics:

- Induced by a postural maneuver (Dix-Hallpike or Barany maneuver) with the abnormal side of the head hanging down
- Latency of onset of nystagmus of 3 seconds to 10 seconds

Table 4.6 Nystagmus: Differentiating Central From Peripheral With Barany Maneuver

Type	Appearance	Latency	Duration	Fatigability	Localization
Central	Multiple directions, may be vertical	Unusual	Persistent	Unusual	Brainstem or cerebellum
Peripheral	Horizontal or torsional	Usual	Brief	Usual	Semicircular canals

- Nystagmus duration only 15 seconds and then the response fatigues
- Unidirectional
- Etiology: benign positional vertigo (labyrinthine concretions)

Central nystagmus—characteristics:

- Multidirectional
- Not inhibited by fixation
- Vertical (upbeat or downbeat) direction
- Dysconjugate nystagmus—nystagmus present in one eye only or of different amplitudes in each eye
- May have a rotatory component
- Neighborhood signs on neurological examination (Rule: Everything in neurology is based on the company you keep.)
- Etiology: brainstem infarction, tumor, cerebellar disease, multiple sclerosis

Caveats

- Drugs (e.g., anticonvulsants) may produce a central type of nystagmus.
- Rotatory nystagmus is typical (but *not* pathognomonic) of a peripheral lesion.

4. Common Etiologies—Difficult to Differentiate

Vestibular neuronitis (overlap with labyrinthitis)

- Etiology unclear? possible postviral syndrome
- Symptoms—vertigo, peripheral nystagmus, nausea, and vomiting
- Associated tinnitus or hearing loss is not characteristic
- Lesion presumably peripheral
- Resolves gradually over 4 days to 10 days

Ménière disease (endolymphatic hydrops)

- Vertigo (often with nausea, vomiting, and nystagmus)
- Tinnitus (variable, may crescendo over minutes to hours, and persist days to weeks)
- Hearing loss: fluctuating but progressive

Cerebellar infarction

- May very closely mimic acute labyrinthitis
- Symptoms—vertigo, nausea, and vomiting
- Nystagmus is *not* peripheral but rather is usually direction-changing (central)
- Symmetrical caloric responses on electronystagmography (ENG) (i.e., no canal paresis)

- Ataxia of the limbs may be entirely absent
- Very early stages of cerebellar hemorrhage may be similar (but this situation can deteriorate rapidly because the hemorrhage may act as a space-occupying lesion in a very restricted area causing impaired alertness)

Nonvestibular causes of dizziness

- New glasses, particularly with astigmatism correction
- After acute oculomotor paralysis
- Multiple sensory system disease [e.g., older diabetic with peripheral neuropathy, decreased visual acuity, and impaired hearing (multisensory dizziness)]
- Chronic anxiety
- Hyperventilation

F. SPINAL CORD COMPRESSION

There is a relatively short list of *neurological emergencies*. The CNS emergencies are coma, stroke, and status epilepticus. In the peripheral nervous system (PNS), the most common emergencies are acute inflammatory polyradiculoneuropathy (otherwise known as Guillain-Barré syndrome) and spinal cord compression.

1. Causes of Spinal Cord Compression

- Abscess
- Hematoma
- Trauma
- Vascular malformation
- Metastasis

Extradural compression of the spinal cord may occur secondary to multiple causes including abscess, hematoma, vertebral fracture with dislocation, and vascular malformation but the most common cause by far is metastasis.

2. Primary Sources of Metastases That Cause Spinal Cord Compression

- Lung
- Breast
- Prostate
- Lymphoma
- Kidney
- Myeloma

Metastases to the spine causing symptoms during life occur in 5% to 10% of all patients with carcinoma. A high index of suspicion followed by thorough investigation is mandatory in the evaluation of back pain in a cancer patient in order to avert a devastating outcome. A vertebral body metastasis with secondary epidural spinal cord compression ultimately results in quadriplegia or paraplegia. Adequate technology is currently available to diagnose and treat metastatic disease to the spine.

3. Pathophysiology

- Lesions causing spinal cord compression result in neurological deficits due to mechanical compression of neural tissues
- Edema (increases the degree of tissue distortion and disrupts cellular connections)
- Ischemia (from blockage of nutrient arteries and draining veins)

4. Clinical Spectrum

Clinical presentation

- Time course and pattern:
  - Rapid progression to maximal deficit in less than 48 hours (30% of patients)
  - Subacute neurological deterioration over 7 days to 10 days (60% of patients)
  - Insidious onset over 4 months to 6 months

- Pain:
  - Focal bone pain
  - Radicular pain (from tumor extension and encroachment on spinal roots)

- Bladder and bowel dysfunction:
  - Overflow incontinence
  - Constipation
  - Late sign/poor prognosis for recovery of ambulation

All types of tumors have been reported to metastasize to the spinal region but lung, breast, prostate, lymphoma, kidney, and myeloma represent the majority. Lung cancer in men and carcinoma of the breast in women are the most common sources. In breast cancer patients a 20% autopsy incidence of spinal metastases has been documented.

Three predominant patterns of symptom progression may be differentiated based on the time course. Some patients (30%) present acutely with rapid progression to maximal neurological deficit in less than 48 hours. Subacute neurological deterioration over 7 days to 10 days is seen most frequently (60%). Diagnostic dilemmas are posed by the remaining 10% of individuals whose symptoms develop insidiously over a 4 month to 6 month period.

Pain is the most common initial presenting symptom by far in patients with metastatic spinal disease. Because 85% of lesions involve bone, early focal bone pain with tenderness to percussion of the spine is the rule. Back pain in a cancer patient should immediately alert the physician to the possibility of an underlying metastatic lesion. Pain produced by bony vertebral disease is focal and arises from stretched and disrupted nerve endings in the periosteum, synovial membranes, anterior and posterior longitudinal ligaments, and the annulus fibrosis of the intervertebral disc. Tumor may later extend and encroach upon the spinal roots producing more ominous radicular pain. Radicular pain occurs in a dermatomal distribution corresponding to the compressed nerve roots and at times is radiating in nature, simulating a herniated intervertebral disc. Radicular pain is worse at night when the spinal column extends to its maximal length and is exacerbated by movement, coughing, or sneezing.

Pain may be insidious, lasting for months or for far briefer duration, but is invariably followed by signs of motor impairment. Subtle weakness may be difficult to detect because of overlying pain and may be misinterpreted by the patient as stiffness or incoordination.

Bowel and bladder dysfunction, characterized by overflow incontinence and constipation, generally occur late in the natural history of spinal cord compression, often in conjunction with quadriplegia or paraplegia. Bladder and bowel impairment forebode a poor prognosis for recovery of ambulation regardless of the treatment modality employed. A notable exception is the early sphincter disturbance seen with T12 through L1 lesions compressing the conus medullaris.

5. Cervical Cord Compression: Common Signs and Symptoms

- Focal bone pain
- Radicular pain in arms
- Decreased biceps reflex
- Weakness of forearm flexion
- Increased tone and reflexes in legs
- Bilateral Babinski signs
- Late: forearm and hand weakness, paraplegia, bowel and bladder dysfunction

6. Conus Medullaris Compression (Figure 4.17)

- Focal bone pain
- Flaccid urinary and rectal sphincters
- Early bowel and bladder dysfunction
- *Saddle* anesthesia = decreased pain and temperature S2 through S5 distribution

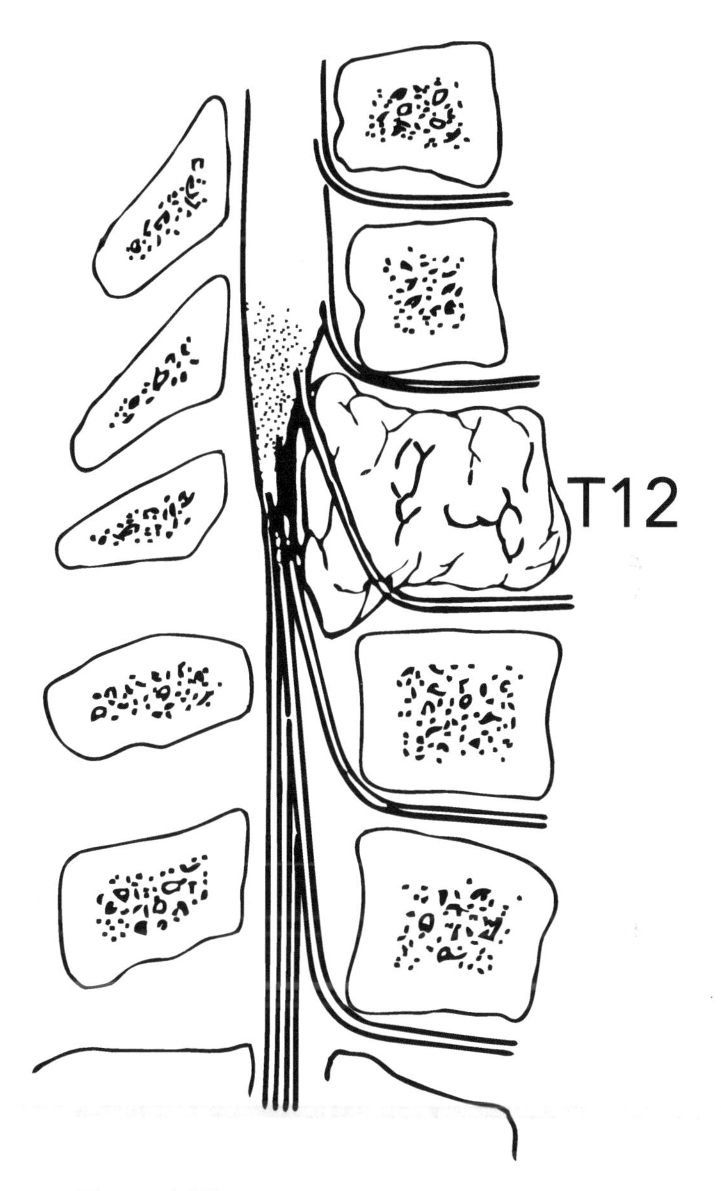

Figure 4.17 Compression of the conus medullaris.

7. Cauda Equina Compression (Figure 4.18)

- Focal bone pain
- Asymmetric radicular pain in legs
- Asymmetric hyporeflexia and weakness in legs
- Late: flaccid paraplegia, areflexia, and incontinence

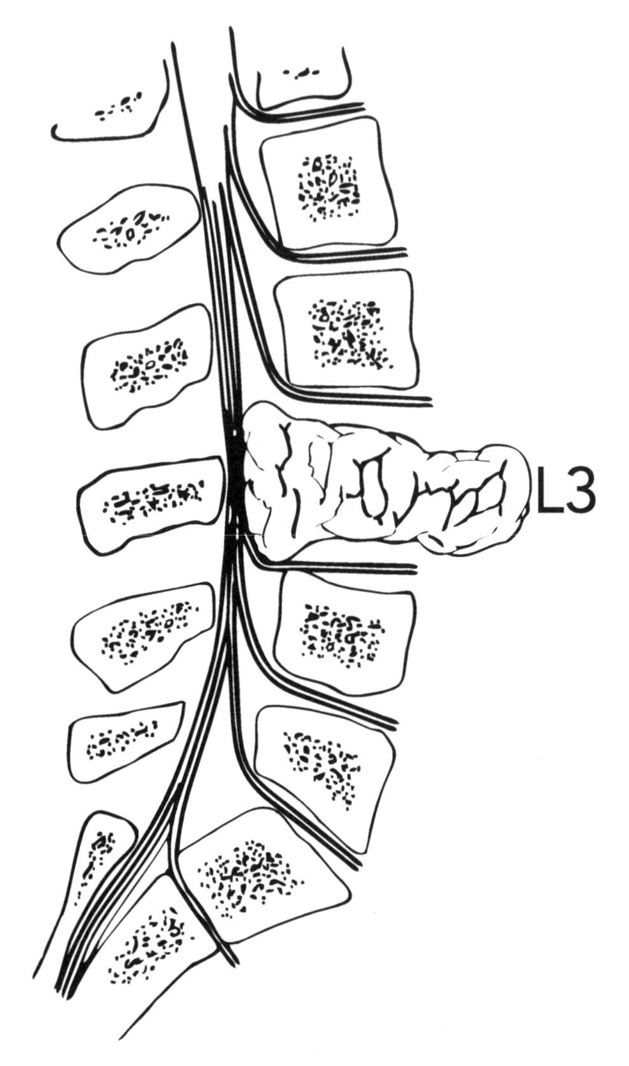

Figure 4.18 Compression of the cauda equina.

8. Summary

Epidural compression of the spinal cord by metastatic tumor occurs in 5% to 10% of patients with malignancy and contributes to morbidity. Detection is facilitated by an understanding of the underlying pathophysiology and the clinical syndromes produced by lesions at various levels of the spinal column.

A complaint of back pain in a patient with cancer should alert the physician to the possibility of an underlying metastatic lesion and impending paralysis. The need for early diagnosis and treatment cannot be overemphasized in a patient with spinal cord compression from any cause.

G. AUTONOMIC NERVOUS SYSTEM

Overview: The autonomic nervous system (ANS) enables, modulates, and controls the automatic functions we take for granted during day-to-day life—until something goes awry. The following are under unconscious control: heart rate, respiration, digestion, pupillary size, salivation, perspiration, urination.

There are two basic ANS divisions: sympathetic and parasympathetic.

1. Sympathetic Nervous System

The cerebral locus is the hypothalamus

- The oculosympathetic pathway—starting in the hypothalamus, extending down into the upper cervical spinal cord, and ascending to the superior cervical ganglion and the eye—is completely uncrossed.
- A lesion of this pathway leads to Horner syndrome
  - Pupillary miosis (small ipsilateral pupil)
  - Ptosis (droopy lid of the ipsilateral eye)
  - Anhidrosis (lack of sweating, and hence dry skin, of the ipsilateral face) (Figure 4.19)

Spinal cord segments T1 through L2 provide sympathetic nerves

- Typically short preganglionic axons and long postganglionic axons
- Cell bodies of the preganglionic neurons are in the lateral horn of the spinal cord (interomediolateral cell columns) from T1 through L2
- Postsynaptic ganglia can be:
  - Paravertebral ganglia—on either side of the vertebral bodies
  - Prevertebral ganglia—celiac ganglion, superior mesenteric ganglion, inferior mesenteric ganglion

2. Parasympathetic Nervous System

- Originates from CNs III, VII, IX, and X and sacral nerves S2 through S4
- Typically long preganglionic axons and short postganglionic axons
- The cranial nerve parasympathetic axons synapse on either the ciliary, pterygopalatine, otic, or submandibular ganglia
- CN X, the wandering vagus nerve, carries parasympathetic outflow to the visceral organs above the level of the splenic flexure
- The pelvic splanchnic nerves control the bladder, ureters, urinary sphincter, anal sphincter, uterus, prostate, and genitalia/sexual function

3. Visceral Sensory Afferents

- Sensory information from the viscera informs the ANS
- Allow for monitoring of blood oxygen, carbon dioxide, and glucose

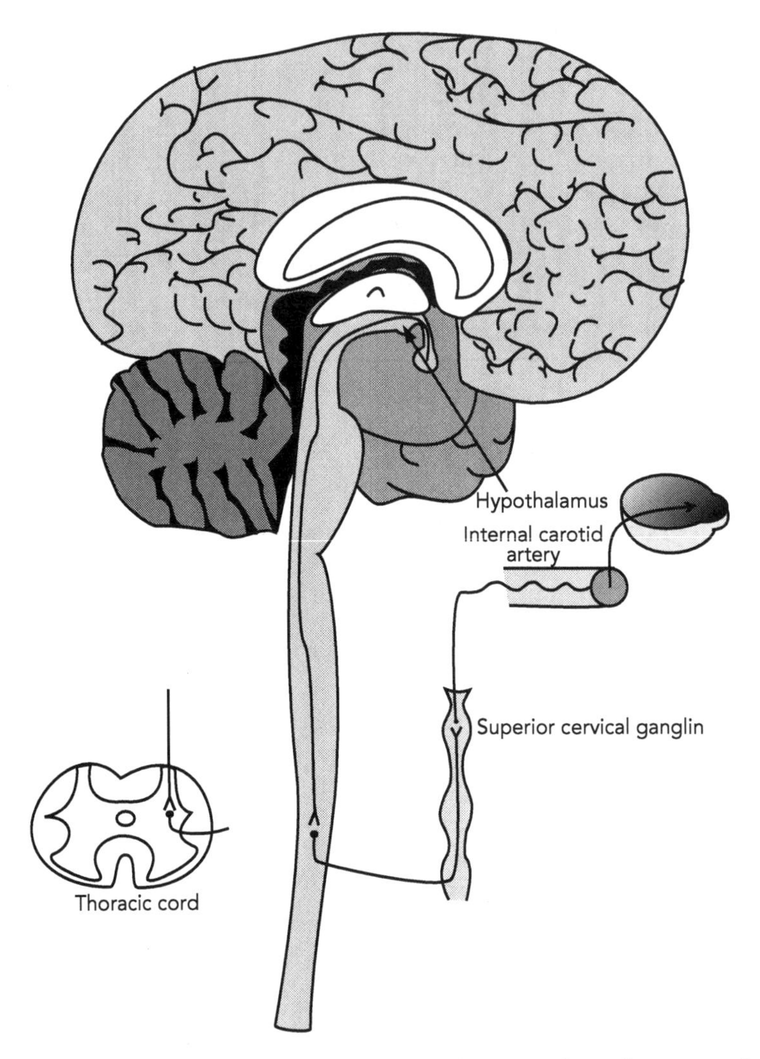

Figure 4.19 Pathway of the oculosympathetic track. A lesion results in ipsilateral Horner syndrome: miosis, ptosis, and anhidrosis.

- Allow for monitoring arterial BP
- Allow for monitoring the chemical composition of the gastrointestinal contents

4. Special Application: Neurourology

Overview: the bladder functions to store urine and expel it at the appropriate time.

The detrusor muscle, a smooth muscle, is the muscle of the bladder. Urine is expelled by contraction of the detrusor muscle and opening of the internal and external urethral sphincters.

The internal urethral sphincter is under autonomic control; the external urethral sphincter is under voluntary control.

Bladder innervation (Figure 4.20)

- Motor input *to* the bladder and urethra:
  - Parasympathetic
    - Preganglionic cell bodies in detrusor nucleus in intermediolateral cell column of the spinal cord (S2–S4)
    - Preganglionic fibers exit the spinal cord as the pelvic splanchnic nerves
    - Fibers synapse in pelvic ganglia located in detrusor muscle and connective tissue of the pelvis
    - Short postganglionic fibers innervate detrusor muscle
  - Somatic
    - Begins in anterior horn cells S2 through S4: the pudendal nucleus or nucleus of Onufrowicz, also known as Onuf
    - Axons form the pudendal nerve
    - Innervates the external urethral sphincter for voluntary control of urination
  - Sympathetic
    - Cell bodies are located in the L1, L2 intermediolateral cell column
    - Preganglionic fibers synapse in paravertebral and preaortic sympathetic ganglia
    - Innervates internal urethral sphincter and smooth muscle of bladder

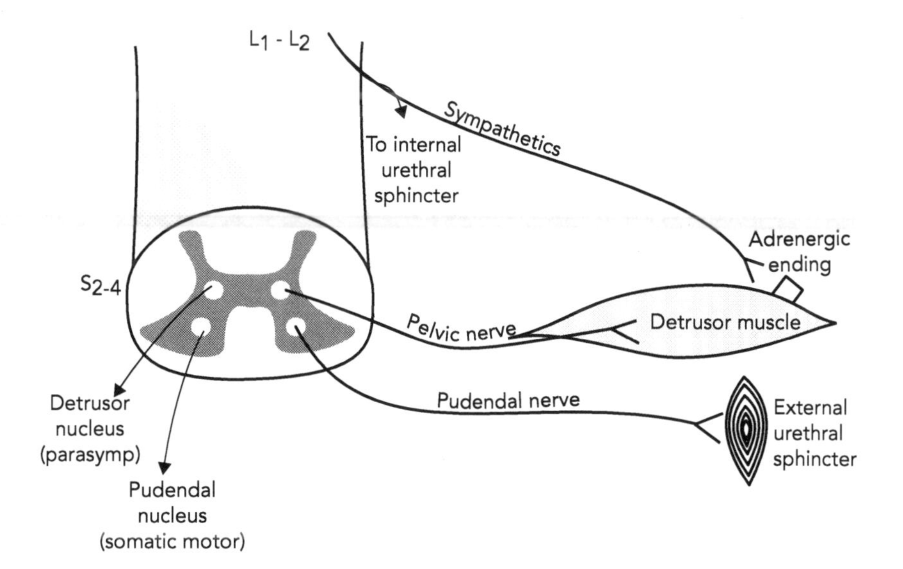

Figure 4.20 Innervation of bladder and urethra.

- Sensory input *from* the bladder and urethra:
  - Parasympathetic
    - Follows pelvic nerves
    - Ascends in lateral column adjacent to lateral spinothalamic tract and in posterior columns to cerebellum, thalamus, and cerebral cortex
    - Mediates sensations to pain, temperature, fullness, and desire to void
  - Somatic
    - Muscle spindle afferents travel in pudendal nerves
    - Synapses S1 through S3 and ascends in posterior columns
    - Modulates tone in external sphincter of bladder
  - Sympathetic
    - Provides vague sensation of pain due to vesicle overdistention
    - Travels with hypogastric nerves
    - Enters dorsal root of levels T6 through L2 to synapse on intermediolateral cell column

Innervation of urethra

- Stretching of urethra causes increased firing of muscle spindles.
- These afferents synapse on the pudendal (Onuf) nucleus creating a reflex arc. Increased firing of the pudendal nucleus tightens the external urethral sphincter.

Micturition—here's what happens

- Bladder filling stretches smooth muscle fibers, causing the detrusor to contract autonomously once the bladder fills past a volume of 150 mL to 200 mL in adults.
- With each contraction, sensory neurons in the detrusor muscle send a burst of signal back to the spinal cord, which is perceived as urgency to void.
- At a normal capacity of 350 mL to 500 mL and in the appropriate situation the voiding reflex is initiated.
- Stretch receptors in the bladder wall *excite* the detrusor nucleus (contracting the detrusor muscle of the bladder) and *inhibit* the pudendal nucleus (relaxing the external urethral sphincter), causing voiding.
- Efferent neural discharges from the brainstem micturition center continue to stimulate the detrusor nucleus until voiding is complete.
- There is also an important role for recurrent inhibition in the sacral spinal cord. There is negative feedback from detrusor motor neurons, via Renshaw cells, onto the bladder. This is influenced by the brainstem and cerebellum, and allows for the physiological performance of specific visceral reflexes separately (i.e., micturition, defecation, and sexual function).

Central pathways controlling micturition (Figure 4.21)

- Cerebrum to pontine micturition center
  - Inhibition until suitable time to void
  - Allows for voluntary initiation and interruption of voiding

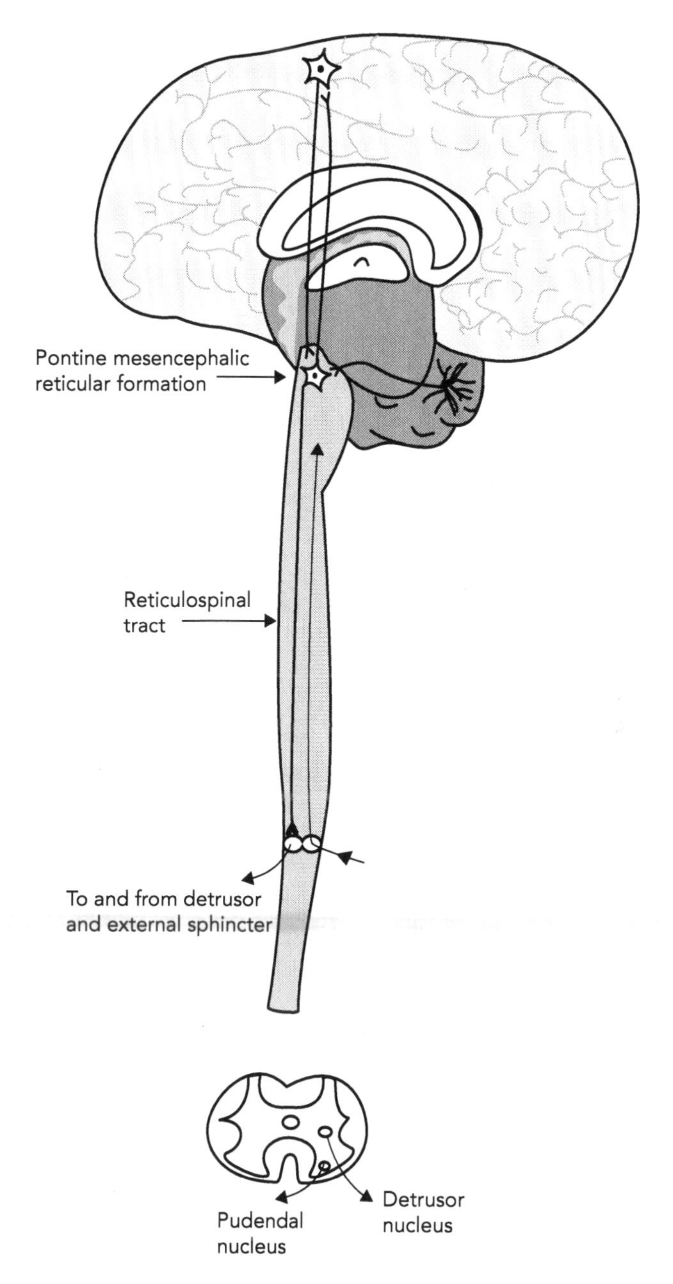

Figure 4.21 Central control of bladder function.

    - Input from: medial frontal lobes; thalamus; red nucleus, subthalamic nucleus, substantia nigra; cerebellum
- Brainstem to sacral gray
    - Provides for complete voiding
    - Descending innervation to detrusor nucleus in sacral cord via reticulospinal tracts

A neurogenic bladder can be overactive (spastic) or underactive (flaccid), and in either case lead to urinary incontinence. The spastic bladder, in general, localizes to an upper motor neuron lesion and a flaccid bladder localizes to a lower motor neuron lesion.

5

Special Applications of Neuro-Logic: Neuropsychiatry

Lorin M. Scher, MD and Julia B. Frank, MD

Although psychiatric disorders are currently diagnosed without reference to anatomy or particular lesions, many elements of psychopathology are associated with dysregulation in areas of the neocortex and the limbic system. These areas are linked by networks of neurons that release and respond to particular neurotransmitters, particularly the monoamines dopamine, norepinephrine, and serotonin.

A. ANATOMY OF NEUROPSYCHIATRIC DISORDERS

The *DSM-5* (*Diagnostic and Statistical Manual of Mental Disorders,* 5th edition) of the American Psychiatric Association (2013) classifies disorders based on symptoms that patients report (e.g., hallucinations) or symptoms that others observe (e.g., delusions). The disorders are also based on patterns of behavior—including neurovegetative behavior such as sleep and psychomotor retardation, or agitation—and stereotypic patterns of autonomic activity (e.g., the fight-or-flight response including panic). By design, the diagnostic criteria for most disorders do *not* require the presence of objective neurological findings. Although the psychiatric syndromes as currently defined do not point to lesions or damage in precise anatomic locations, they do involve dysfunction in specifiable, albeit relatively broad, brain areas and circuits. This discussion focuses on the frontal lobe and associated subcortical structures that are the areas most involved in the pathogenesis of many psychiatric syndromes.

1. Frontal Lobe

The frontal lobe is the largest lobe of the human brain, representing almost 33% of the total volume of the cerebral cortex.

- Functional and in vivo metabolic imaging techniques, such as fMRI (functional magnetic resonance imaging) and positron emission tomography (PET), have transformed behavioral neurology (which overlaps with much of psychopathology) from a lesional field—where localization is based on neurological deficits identified following an acquired lesion—to a functional field, where physiological malfunctioning can be observed.
- Compared to primates and other species, the human frontal lobes are massive in size and have unique cytoarchitecture. Chimpanzees, dogs, and cats have 17%, 7%, and 3.5% of human frontal lobe volume, respectively. Pyramidal cells in the human prefrontal cortex are more complex, with more spines and branching than those in other primate species.
- Three parallel, segregated, reciprocal circuits connect the dorsolateral, orbitomedial, and anterior cingulate regions of the prefrontal cortex with limbic structures, including discrete areas of the thalamus and the caudate nucleus. These circuits mediate executive functions.
- In neuroscience research (both human and animal), executive functions are measured by performance on tasks that require planning, initiating, maintaining, and self-checking.
- More broadly defined, executive functions encompass the human capacities for abstraction, sequencing, focused attention, creative problem solving, motivated behavior, and the ability to respond to changing environments. They create unique human capacities to integrate information from various sources, plan and make decisions, and generate new thoughts.

2. The Prefrontal Cortex

- Dorsolateral area (Brodmann areas 9, 10, and 46)
- Orbitofrontal area
- Anterior cingulate (medial) area

For reorientation, we return to Figure 2.2 in Chapter 2 (here Figure 5.1), showing the Brodmann areas over the lateral cortex (Brodmann areas 9, 10, 11, and 46 are shown; area 24 would be deep and medial).

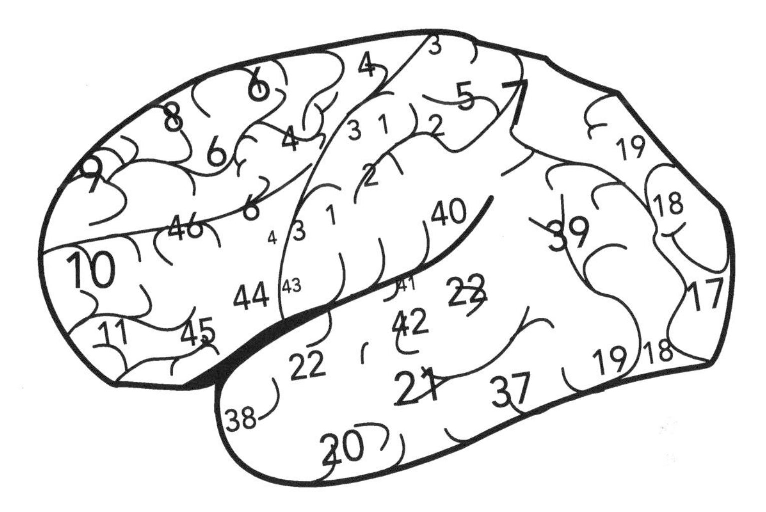

Figure 5.1 Brodmann areas of the brain.

Although clinically distinct, the dorsolateral, orbitofrontal, and medial cingulate syndromes of the prefrontal cortex all influence the ability to either register or to filter stimuli (afferent functions), an essential step in the ability to pursue goal-directed behavior (efferent functions). Figure 5.2 demonstrates more detail of the prefrontal cortex.

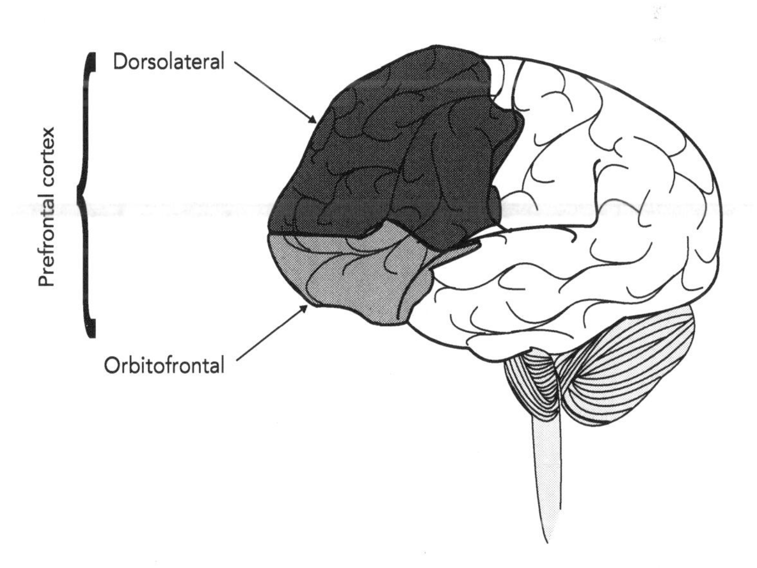

Figure 5.2 The dorsolateral and orbitofrontal areas of the prefrontal cortex.

Importance of the prefrontal cortex in psychiatry

Early interest in the prefrontal cortex dates historically to the bizarre accident in 1848 of Phineas Gage, who survived an explosion that drove an iron rod through his prefrontal cortex. Despite continued normal intelligence, he changed from being conscientious, serious, and motivated to childlike, immature, and socially inappropriate.

- Dorsolateral prefrontal area:
  - Afferents: dorsomedial nucleus of the thalamus, limbic system via cingulate gyrus and orbital cortices, hypothalamus
  - Efferents: reciprocal connections with the thalamus and head of the caudate from the frontal-subcortical circuit
  - Dorsolateral lesion: abulic or apathetic syndrome, characterized by inattentiveness, hypokinesis, and impoverished affect; inability to maintain goal-directed behavior, focus, or sustained effort; pseudodepression: react to environmental stimuli with loss of volitional control of behavior
  - Relation to psychopathology: depression

- Orbitofrontal area:
  - Afferents: dorsomedial nucleus of thalamus, hypothalamus, amygdala, uncinate fasciculus, sensory cortex, frontal association cortex.
  - Efferents: reciprocal connections to afferent regions, caudate nucleus, globus pallidus, and substantia nigra: the orbitofrontal-subcortical circuit. These operate semi-independently of the dorsolateral-basal circuit previously described. Lesion studies indicate that this region regulates social rules of conduct (considering consequences of behavior, concern for the feelings of others).
  - Orbitofrontal lesions: frontal convexity syndrome, also known as the euphoric syndrome: hyperactivity, excitable or exaggerated affect, irritability, emotional shallowness, childish humor, sexual disinhibition, diminished empathy, decreased ability to assess risk or limit behavior based on consequences. Trauma, stroke, hydrocephalus, compressive (e.g., meningioma) and intrinsic tumors (e.g., glioma) are among the neurological etiologies of this syndrome.
  - Relation to psychopathy: patients with mania and some forms of schizophrenia show similar deficits.

- Anterior cingulate cortex:
  - Afferents: receive connections from hippocampus, dorsomedial nucleus of the thalamus, hypothalamus, amygdala, and sensory association cortex.
  - Efferents: project to the nucleus accumbens, globus pallidus, substantia nigra, and dorsomedial nucleus of the thalamus.

- Anterior cingulate lesions: apathy related to loss of motivation that is also mediated by projecting dopaminergic afferent input.
- Relation to psychopathology: panic disorder may involve activation of the connection between the amygdala and the interior cingulate gyrus. Stimuli that would normally be ignored instead command attention and the person reacts with alarm.

Frontal lobe dysfunction and psychiatric illness

- Schizophrenia:

  The cognitive and personality related (negative) symptoms of schizophrenia (which may exist separately from the psychotic or positive symptoms) involve frontal lobe dysfunction.

  - Patients with schizophrenia may perform poorly on neuropsychological tests that measure frontal lobe function (Wisconsin Card Sorting Test, verbal fluency, design fluency, tower test).
  - fMRI studies have found decreased activation in prefrontal gray matter, and a loss of the normal right greater than left asymmetry in activation of the superior prefrontal cortex.
  - Other studies, for example, SPECT (single photon emission computed tomography), have shown that patients with schizophrenia have both decreased blood flow and reduced metabolic activity in the frontal lobes during a resting state.

- Mood disorders:

  - Depression and bipolar affective disorder are associated with frontal lobe, limbic, and hypothalamic-pituitary axis (HPA) dysfunction.
  - Dorsolateral and orbitofrontal apathetic syndromes, including inattentiveness, hypokinesis (psychomotor retardation), impoverished speech, and decreased motivation, are common symptoms of depression. Depression also involves diminished capacity to experience pleasure (anhedonia), related to dysregulated functioning of the mesolimbic pathway connecting the ventral tegmental area, ventral striatum (nucleus accumbens), and medial prefrontal cortex.
  - Orbitofrontal dysfunction produces hyperactivity, euphoria, irritability, and mood lability, as seen in hypomania and mania.

- Obsessive compulsive disorder (OCD):

  - Clinical symptoms of disturbing thoughts of guilt or distress over a planned action (obsessions) reflect disturbed executive function.
  - Conscious repetitive behaviors (compulsions) develop to relieve the anxiety generated by the obsessions.
  - fMRI shows increased metabolic activity and perfusion in the orbitofrontal cortex, caudate nucleus, thalamus, and anterior cingulate gyrus (hyperfrontality) in OCD.

- Panic disorder:
    - Anterior cingulate gyrus: reduced filtering of incoming information
    - Orbitomedial prefrontal cortex: negative emotional response to input
    - Excessive arousal with imbalance of sympathetic/parasympathetic activity

- Pain disorders:
    - Depression, anxiety disorders, and somatoform disorders may involve pain, either without known lesions or in excess of what would be expected from a lesion (central sensitization). Patients may devote excessive attention to pain, interpret pain as unduly threatening, or associate it with particular memories.
    - The CNS (central nervous system) matrix that processes and responds to painful stimuli includes primary and secondary somatosensory areas, the insula, anterior cingulate gyrus, and prefrontal cortices as well as the thalamus, amygdala, cerebellum, and brainstem.

- Posttraumatic stress disorder:
    - Neurochemicals released in response to severe stress affect the structure and function of particular brain areas, especially the hippocampus (normally the site of declarative memory), amygdala, and medial prefrontal cortex.
    - Cardinal symptoms of intrusive recollection, flashbacks, nightmares, and selective or fluctuating amnesia represent abnormally encoded fearful memories.

- Addictions:
    - Drug-related cues stimulate the mesolimbic pathway (cingulate gyrus/nucleus accumbens circuit), generating motivation to use the rewarding substance.
    - Lateral orbitofrontal cortex, which usually triggers consideration of context and risk, has reduced function and user does not consider consequences of drug use.

B. NEUROTRANSMITTER SYSTEMS

The brain areas implicated in many psychiatric disorders are linked by networks of neurons originating in the brainstem. Each neuron that originates in a particular area releases only one monoamine neurotransmitter. The neurotransmitter networks may function independently, in parallel, or modulate each other (Figure 5.3). These overlapping and discrete functions explain the selective actions of drugs that affect the functions of particular neurotransmitters, through a variety of mechanisms (e.g., blockade of reuptake, potentiating release by altering feedback, changing the expression of genes that regulate receptor function).

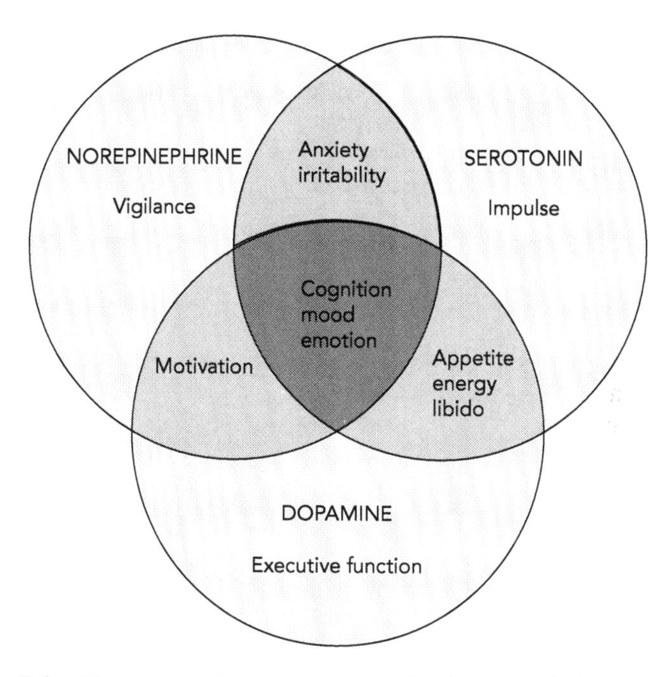

Figure 5.3 Neurotransmitter systems in the brain and their overlapping roles.

1. Dopaminergic Systems

Nigrostriatal

- Project from substantia nigra to corpus striatum (caudate and putamen).
- Receptors are both D1 and D2.
- Blocking D2 with traditional antipsychotics (e.g., haloperidol) causes extrapyramidal side effects (EPS), including Parkinsonism (mask-like facies, cogwheel rigidity, pill-rolling tremor), akathisia (subjective restlessness), and dystonia.

Mesolimbic

- Project from ventral tegmentum of the midbrain to the nucleus accumbens.
- Involved in sensation of reward and pathogenesis of addiction.
- Malfunctions in depression, with lost capacity for pleasure, producing anhedonia.

- Antipsychotic drugs may induce dysphoria and anhedonia by blocking mesolimbic dopaminergic pathways. Blockade of these receptors also contributes to the reduction of manic symptoms by dopamine blocking drugs.

Mesocortical

- Project from the ventral tegmentum of the midbrain to the prefrontal, cingulate, and entorhinal cortices.
- Regulate executive functions: planning, sequencing, abstraction.
- Shape aspects of personality, including motivation, impulsiveness, self-control, social judgment.
- Disruption contributes to psychotic symptoms in schizophrenia, delirium, dementia, depression.

2. Dopamine Hypothesis: Pathophysiology of Psychotic or Positive Symptoms in Schizophrenia

- Schizophrenia affects 1% of people; incidence in men equals incidence in women. Disorder reflects interplay of many genes of small effect. Often associated with alcohol or illicit drug use (especially cocaine and phencyclidine).
- Functional excess of dopamine.
- Dopamine receptor blockers have antipsychotic activity, and dopaminergic agonists may induce psychotic symptoms.
- All effective antipsychotics block the D2 receptors that are especially plentiful in the mesocortical pathway. Serotonergic neurons parallel dopaminergic neurons in this pathway, allowing for second-generation antipsychotics that block the activity of D2 receptors partly by regulating serotonin but leave other dopamine pathways relatively intact, thereby causing fewer movement side effects.

3. Serotonergic System

- Precursor is tryptophan.
  - Dietary variations in tryptophan affect brain serotonin levels.
  - Diet low in tryptophan causes irritability and hunger.
  - Diet high in tryptophan induces sleep, relieves anxiety, and increases sense of well-being.
  - Metabolized to 5-HIAA (5-hydroxyindoleacetic acid), which can be measured in CSF (cerebrospinal fluid).
- Serotonergic neurons project widely throughout the brain, originating in the upper pons and midbrain (the median dorsal raphe nuclei) and projecting to cerebral cortex, basal ganglia, limbic system, hypothalamus, cerebellum, and brainstem.

  - Serotonin acts as a general modulator, regulating noradrenergic and dopaminergic processes, as well as hypothalamic and spinal cord function. Serotonergic action on the hypothalamus regulates vegetative functions such as sleep, appetite, energy, and libido.
  - Serotonin also modulates cognitive function in the neocortex.
  - Serotonin plays a major role in psychiatric disorders, particularly anxiety, depression, and psychosis. Decreased levels of serotonin and 5-HIAA (the major serotonin metabolite) are found in the brains and CSF of depressed patients, and increasing the availability of serotonin often alleviates symptoms of depression. Decreased 5-HIAA in spinal fluid has been associated with suicide and violence, regardless of the primary psychiatric diagnosis.
  - There is, however, no single-neurotransmitter–single-illness relationship. Increasing the availability of norepinephrine and dopamine also relieves depressive symptoms. Dual reuptake inhibitors and selective norepinephrine reuptake inhibitors also relieve depression, anxiety, and sometimes pain.

4. Central Cholinergic System

- Acetylcholine (Ach) projections connect the brainstem and basal forebrain.
  - Brainstem projections stem from the pedunculopontine and laterodorsal tegmental regions, and project to the basal ganglia, thalamus, and hippocampus.
  - Basal forebrain cell bodies extend from the septum, band of Broca, and nucleus basalis of Meynert and project to the thalamus, limbic system, and cerebral cortex.
  - The nucleus basalis of Meynert specifically degenerates in Alzheimer disease, causing widespread deficiency of acetylcholine in the brain.
  - Limbic and neocortical cells deteriorate and eventually die due to the loss of cholinergic input. Drugs that potentiate acetylcholine function slow the progression of Alzheimer dementia, especially in the early stages, before widespread cell death has occurred.
  - Dopamine and acetylcholine have a reciprocal relationship in the nigrostriatal dopamine pathway. In this pathway, dopaminergic neurons make postsynaptic inhibitory connections with cholinergic neurons. When dopamine is available, acetylcholine activity is suppressed. Alternatively, when dopamine is blocked (e.g., with haloperidol), acetylcholine becomes overactive, and hence extrapyramidal symptoms (EPS) (e.g., acute and tardive dyskinesias) are produced. Anticholinergic medications are commonly given with typical antipsychotics to decrease the incidence of EPS.

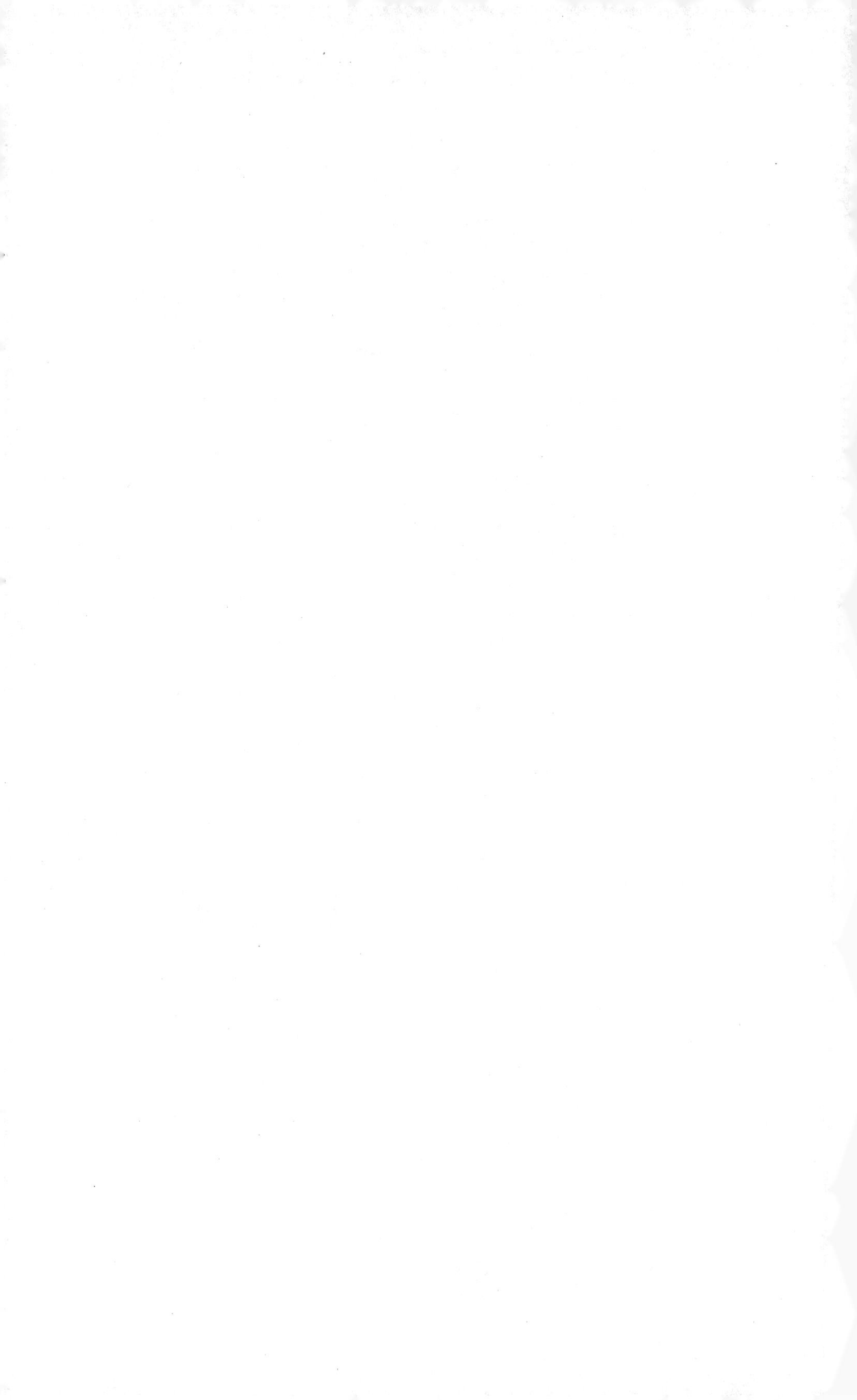

6

The Neurological Examination and Putting It All Together

A discussion of clinical localization is incomplete without some attention to the neurological examination. The neurological examination in particular is recognized as a specialized clinical skill that is dedicated to confirm or deny aspects of the neurological history, and is designed to assist with the localization of a patient's disturbance(s) affecting the nervous system. The examination should include at least five basic areas and should be reported, either in written or oral format, in a logical rostrocaudal order. This promotes the intellectual process of localization.

Begin with *mental status*, then *cranial nerves*, and then include the other elements: *motor, sensory,* and *reflexes*. Testing for cerebellar, balance, and gait should be included, whether as part of the motor exam or as separate components.

A. MENTAL STATUS EXAM

- Check for alertness and orientation multiplied by 4 (person, place, time, and purpose [i.e., What is your name? Where are you? About what time is it? Why are you here?])
- Check for overall knowledge base, attention, concentration, calculations (serial 7s [i.e., start with the number 100 and subtract 7 serially])

- Assess memory functions (recall of three out of three unrelated words after a 5-minute interval)
- Language (fluency, comprehension, repetition, naming)
- Assess mood (patient reports), affect (patient transmits)
- Thought processes (delusional? paranoid? grandiose?)
- Thought content (realistic? delusions? paranoia? ideas of reference?)
- Scales such as the Folstein Mini-Mental Status Examination may be useful

The mini-mental status exam (MMSE) consists of a series of questions testing orientation, registration, attention, recall, and language. A score of 25 or more points (out of 30 points maximum) is effectively normal (intact). Below this, scores can indicate severe (less than or equal to 9 points), moderate (10 points–20 points), or mild (21 points–24 points) cognitive impairment. Mild cognitive impairment (MCI) is a term applied to aging individuals with noticeable cognitive deficits, often in the sphere of memory, that are not of sufficient severity to diagnose dementia. MCI is estimated to affect 10% to 20% of adults age 65 and older.

B. CRANIAL NERVE EXAM

There are 12 cranial nerves (CNs); these are sensory, motor, or both. They can be tested fairly quickly by using the following maneuvers:

CN I—Olfactory nerve: often omitted (unfortunately) but scents can be tested in each nostril.

CN II—Optic nerve: check for pupillary light reflex (afferent arc is mediated by CN II; efferent arc and consensual response are mediated by CN III), visual fields to finger counting, visual acuity, funduscopy. Use the swinging flashlight test: a consensually constricted pupil that then dilates indicates a relative afferent pupillary defect.

CNs III, IV, and VI—Oculomotor, Trochlear, and Abducens nerves: these innervate the extraocular muscles. Test eye movements in all directions of gaze.

CN V—Trigeminal nerve: Check sensation over all three facial innervated regions: V1 (ophthalmic), V2 (maxillary), and V3 (mandibular). This also mediates the afferent arc of the corneal reflex (efferent arc is CN VII) and motor innervation to the masseter muscle, tested by clenching the jaw.

CN VII—Facial nerve: test facial movement with patient asked to demonstrate expressions (i.e., smile, frown, raise eyebrows).

CN VIII—Vestibulocochlear nerve: whisper or rub fingers for sound detection. Expect Weber to show that sound is heard symmetrically via vibrating tuning fork held at the midforehead, and Rinne to show that air conduction is symmetrically greater than bone conduction when the tuning fork is first held on the mastoid process behind the ear and then placed alongside the ear.

CNs IX and X—Glossopharyngeal and Vagus nerves: usually tested together. Check gag reflex (afferent arc is IX, efferent arc is X).

CN XI—Spinal-Accessory nerve: test sternocleidomastoid muscle strength by having patient turn the head to either side against resistance. Also check trapezius strength via shoulder shrug for spinal component.

CN XII—Hypoglossal nerve: check tongue protrusion and lateral movement.

C. MOTOR EXAM

Examine muscles for bulk, tone, and strength. Individualized muscle group strength testing is graded on a scale of 0 to 5 with zero designating not even a flicker of voluntary movement, as follows:

1/5: palpable or visible contraction only
2/5: full range of motion but only with gravity eliminated
3/5: full range of motion but only against gravity
4/5: full range of motion against partial resistance (i.e., decreased strength)
5/5: normal strength against full resistance

Have the person hold out both arms, palms up with eyes closed. This may reveal subtle hemiparesis (weaker arm pronates and drops slightly [pronator drift]).

D. SENSORY EXAM

Check the sensation over the face and extremities to multiple modalities:

- Light touch
- Pain and temperature (broken wooden swab and cold tuning fork are commonly used)
- Vibratory sensation
- Proprioception
- Graphesthesia (palm writing)
- Stereognosia (name object placed in hand with eyes closed)
- Two-point discrimination (identify two objects a similar distribution apart spatially over either side)
- Double simultaneous stimulation (distinguish stimulation with one versus two stimuli)

E. REFLEXES

- Deep tendon reflexes (biceps, triceps, brachioradialis, patellar, Achilles) are graded on a scale:
  - 0—absent
  - Trace—minimally present

- o 1+—hypoactive, may be normal
- o 2+—average/typical
- o 3+—hyperactive, may be normal
- o 4+—sustained with clonus

Check for pathological reflexes, especially the Babinski, where an upgoing great toe—when the foot is stroked along the lateral aspect and then across the dorsum—indicates an upper motor neuron lesion (or, rarely, neuromuscular disorder where the toe flexors are weaker than extensors).

F. GAIT/CEREBELLAR

Check routine gait as well as heel, toe, and tandem gait. Evaluate the base (distance between the feet), stride (length and smoothness), associated swing of the arms, posture, and any adventitious movement or asymmetry. Test finger-to-nose and heel-to-shin performance for cerebellar control of movement. The Romberg is frequently added here, and is formally a test of proprioception when the eyes are closed and the patient then falters.

G. EXAMINATION OF THE COMATOSE PATIENT

The coma examination would be used for an unresponsive patient or a patient suffering a decline in consciousness. This is more focused on brainstem reflexes and is discussed in Chapter 4, Part A. In this case, the examination is sometimes done using the Glasgow Coma Scale (GCS).

The GCS was originally devised to predict the prognosis of patients with brain injuries. It assigns a numerical score in the categories of eye movement, verbal response, and motor response. The GCS is graded as follows:

Eye Response

1. No eye opening
2. Eye opening in response to pain
3. Eye opening to speech
4. Eyes opening spontaneously

Verbal Response

1. No verbal response
2. Incomprehensible sounds/moaning

3. Inappropriate words
4. Confused speech
5. Coherent and appropriate response to questions

Motor Response

1. No motor response
2. Extension to pain (decerebrate response)
3. Abnormal flexion to pain (decorticate response)
4. Flexion/withdrawal to pain
5. Localizes to pain (i.e., purposeful movements toward painful stimuli)
6. Obeys commands

The maximum score that can be obtained on the GCS is a 15 and the minimum is a 3. Mortality is high when the GCS score is a 6 or lower. Although the GCS has limitations in terms of localization, it can be used to predict the relative prognosis of a patient with a traumatic brain injury and to follow a patient serially in an emergency department or intensive care unit setting. There are modified scales for infants and children.

A full coma examination would account for these elements, as explained in Chapter 4, Part A.

Mental Status

1. Alert = maintaining wakefulness, interaction, vigilance
2. Lethargic = patient drifts off when not stimulated
3. Stuporous = patient does not alert even with stimulation
4. Delirium = alternating or fluctuating level of consciousness, during which a patient may be agitated, incoherent, or confused
5. Comatose = no purposeful response to nociceptive stimulation

Respiratory Pattern

1. Hemispheric pattern = Cheyne-Stokes
2. Midbrain pattern = central neurogenic hyperventilation
3. Pontine pattern = apneustic breathing
4. Medullary pattern = ataxic breathing

Pupils

1. Hemispheric = pupils equal, round, reactive to light
2. Midbrain = pupils lose reactivity and dilate
3. Pons = pinpoint pupils
4. Medullary = pupils may be normally reactive in isolated medullary lesions causing coma

Extraocular Movements

1. Assess for gaze deviation
   - Gaze toward the lesion and away from hemiparesis in cortical lesion
   - Gaze away from the lesion and toward the hemiparesis in brainstem lesion
2. Oculocephalic reflex = doll's eyes; move the head and watch the eyes float
3. Oculovestibular reflex = caloric responses; eyes should move toward the ice

Motor

1. Assess for focal deficits
2. Posturing (see Figure 4.6)
   - Decorticate posturing
     - o Upper extremities are flexed; lower extremities are extended
     - o Lesion from the cortex to the midbrain, approximating the level of the red nucleus
     - o "Thumbs up": better prognosis than decerebrate posturing
   - Decerebrate posturing
     - o Upper extremities and lower extremities are extended
     - o Lesion from lower midbrain to pontomedullary junction
     - o "Thumbs down": worse prognosis than decorticate posturing
   - Flaccid paralysis
     - o Lesion below the upper medulla

Index

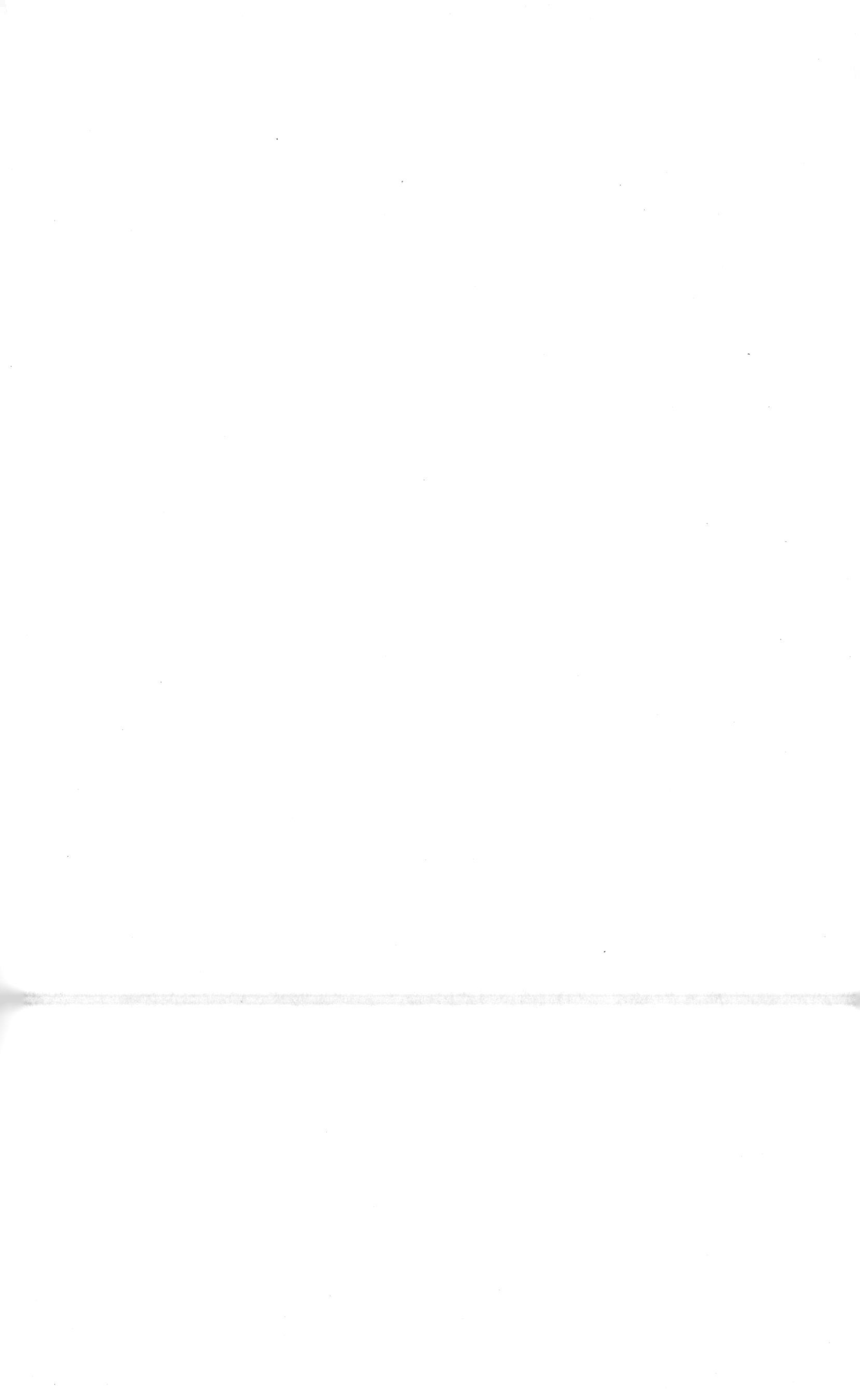

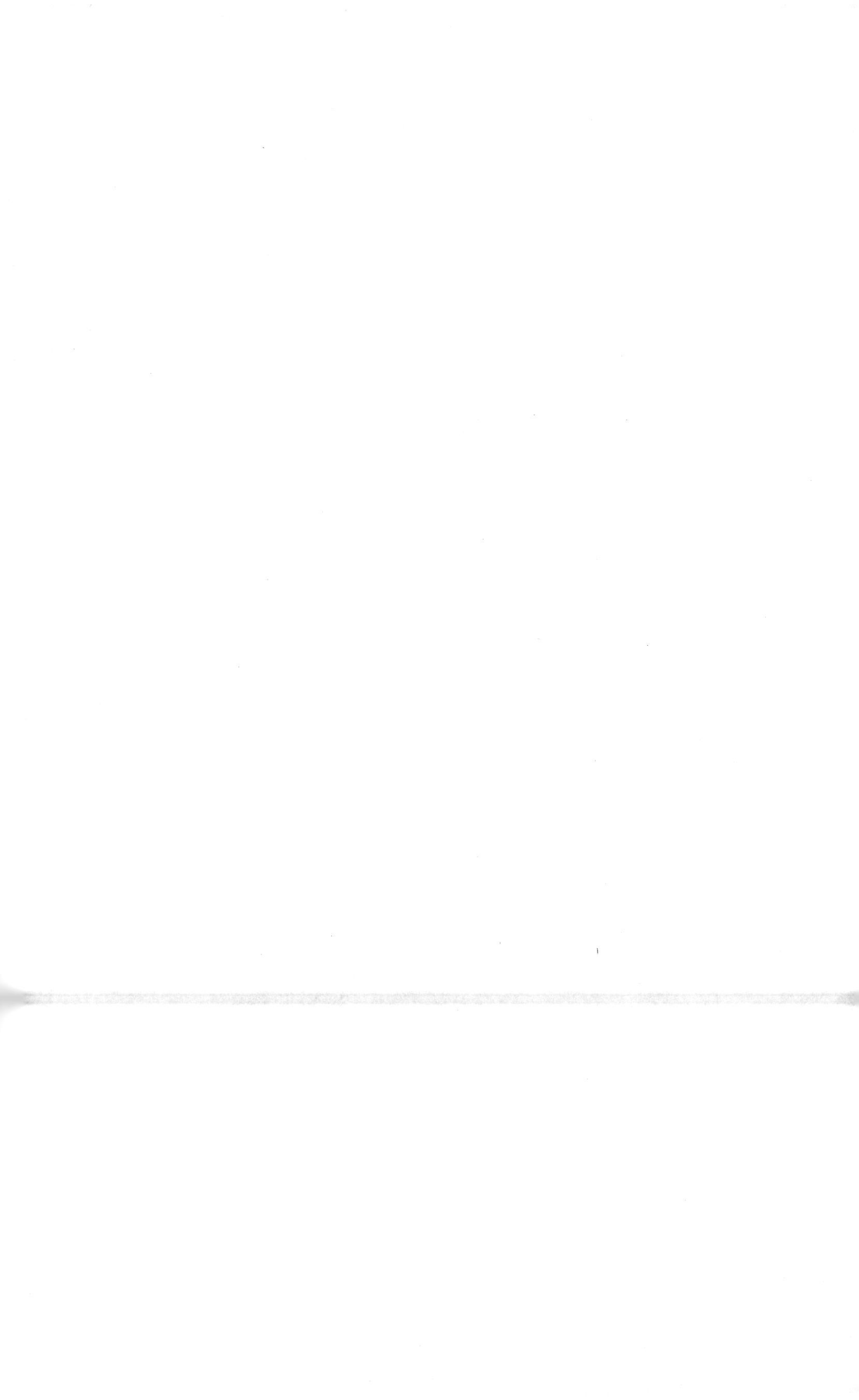

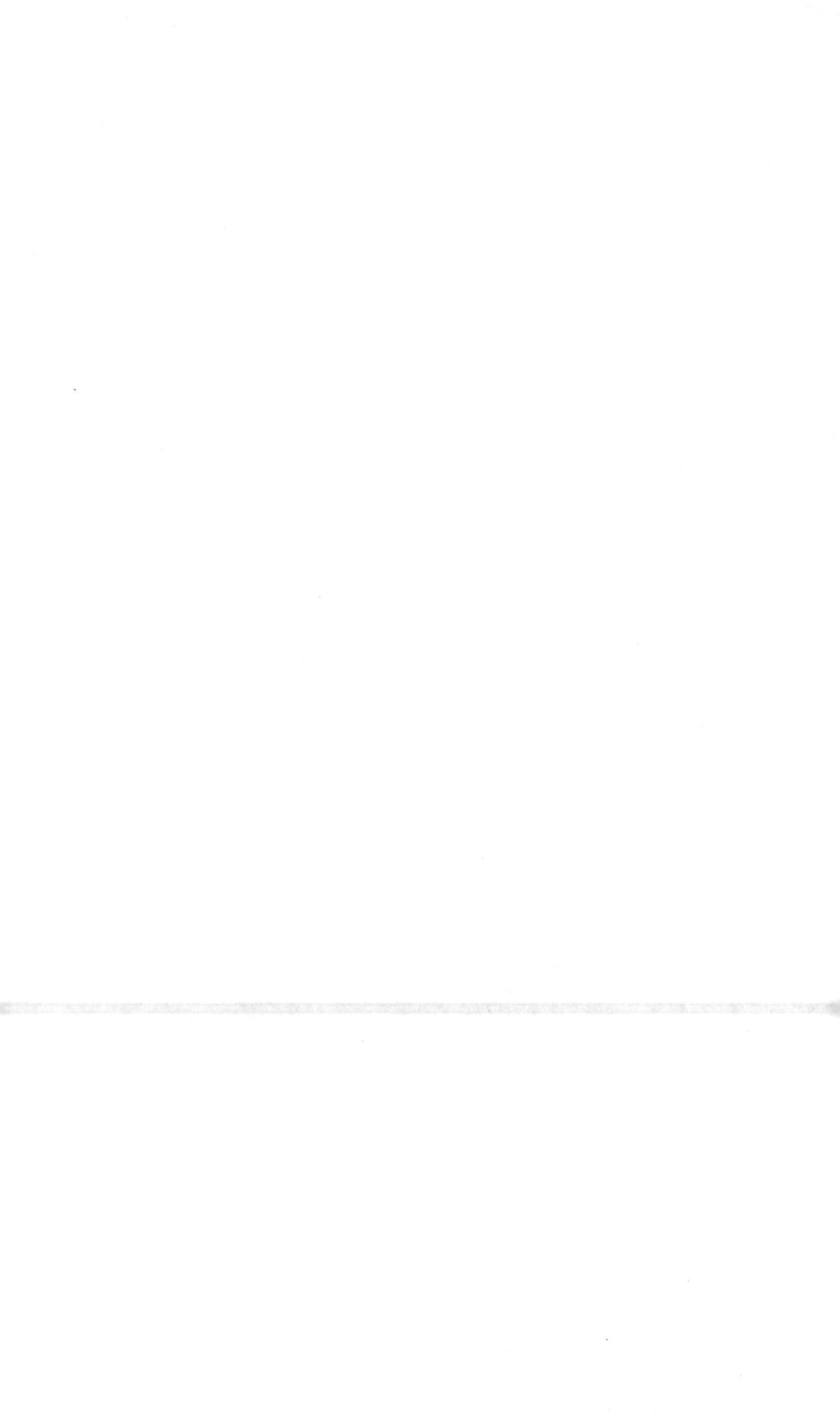